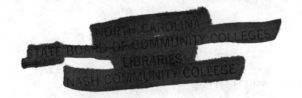
From AIDS to the Internet: Correctional Realities

D1301433

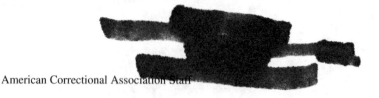

American Correctional Association Staff

Richard L. Stalder, President
James A. Gondles, Jr., Executive Director
Gabriella M. Daley, Director, Communications and Publications
Leslie A. Maxam, Asst. Director, Communications and Publications
Alice Fins, Publications Managing Editor
Michael Kelly, Associate Editor
Sherry Wulfekuhle, Editorial Assistant
Dana M. Murray, Graphics and Production Manager
Traci F. Drake, Graphics and Production Associate
Cover design by Traci F. Drake

Thanks to the staff of *Corrections Today* and *Corrections Compendium* from which many of these articles were adapted.

Printed in the United States of America by Kirby Lithographic Company, Inc., Arlington Virginia

ISBN 1-56991- 110-X
This publication may be ordered from:
American Correctional Association
4380 Forbes Boulevard
Lanham, Maryland 20706-4322
1-800-222-5646

For information on publications and videos available from ACA, contact our worldwide web home page at: http://www.corrections.com/aca.

Library of Congress Cataloging-in-Publication Data
From AIDS to the Internet: Correctional Realities.
        p.   cm.
    ISBN 1-56991-110-X
    1. Criminal justice, Administration of -- United States.
    2. Corrections--United States--Management. 3. Information storage and
    retrieval systems--Criminal justice. Administration of--United States. I.
    American Correctional Association.
    HV9950.F77   1999
    364.6'0973--dc21   98-55315
                                                            CIP

Introduction

Since 1870, the American Correctional Association has dedicated itself to the cause of corrections and correctional effectiveness. Our primary mission is to be of service to correctional professionals, and one of our most important services is to keep people in the profession informed.

The field of corrections currently is facing many pressing issues. Some of these concerns have been around for as long as anybody can remember, such as tuberculosis; others are particular to the last two decades, such as AIDS; while some other issues are relatively new to corrections, such as the use of the Internet. *From AIDS to the Internet: Correctional Realities* addresses these and other topics that impact corrections every day. Assembled from some of the most important articles to appear recently in *Corrections Today*, *Corrections Compendium*, and *The State of Corrections*, this book takes an interesting look at current developments in the areas of healthcare, substance abuse treatment, technology, law, privatization, restorative justice, and media relations.

Corrections is an ever-changing field. Every year we face new challenges, technological breakthroughs, and evolving legal interpretations which demand that we approach our jobs differently. We at the American Correctional Association want correctional professionals to be as informed as possible about what is happening in the field of criminal justice. The twenty-five essays in this book will help do that.

If you are not a member of the American Correctional Association, I urge you to join. If you are already a member, please stay involved with your association so that you may have a hand in advancing and improving corrections. If you would like more information about ACA membership and our publishing program, please contact us at 1-800-ACA-JOIN.

James A. Gondles, Jr.
Executive Director
American Correctional Association

Table of Contents

HIV and TB in Prison:

Increasing Incidence of Infectious Diseases Calls for Aggressive Plan of Action

By Richard Braithwaite, Ph.D.,
Kisha Braithwaite,
and Ronald Poulson, Ph.D.

*I*n addition to the already daunting problems posed by crowding and fiscal stringency, today's correctional administrators and health care professionals must deal with an increasingly ill, troubled, and "graying" inmate population. HIV/AIDS, sexually transmitted diseases, and tuberculosis (TB) represent complex and major communicable diseases for this population. These health and psychosocial problems, including substance abuse and mental illness, are becoming increasingly common among inmates.

Traditionally associated with high-risk sexual activity, drug use, poverty, disenfranchised status, population density, homelessness, and poor access to preventive and primary health care, the health problems of the inmate population pose difficult programmatic and fiscal challenges for correctional policymakers and personnel. Ironically, these concerns also create opportunities and challenges for public health agencies, community-based organizations, and correctional systems to address and improve the health of a particularly underserved and vulnerable segment of society.

Better HIV/AIDS, TB, and sexually transmitted disease-prevention programs, as well as regular medical care, also can benefit society at large, since the majority of inmates return to the community. It would be prudent for inmates to return to their homes armed with prevention knowledge, healthy attitudes, and concepts of appropriate behavior to reduce their risk of infecting others or encountering these communicable diseases.

HIV/AIDS

The past and current behaviors of inmates increase the risk of HIV infection among incarcerated populations. The rate of HIV infection and AIDS is significantly higher among inmates than in the general population. In fact, correctional populations have the highest rates of HIV infection of any public institution. Moreover, previously incarcerated inmates may pose a greater threat of HIV transmission upon release than do other population groups.

Efforts to reduce the incidence of HIV infection among offenders are complex, and pose numerous policy and program-implementation issues for the criminal justice and public health systems. Prison officials acknowledge that sexual intercourse occurs within their facilities. But while condom use is the most effective method of preventing HIV transmission, the distribution of condoms (considered contraband) as a strategy to promote safer sex presents a serious dilemma for prison officials.

Likewise, injection drug use also occurs in prison, but prison officials may be reluctant to provide information on the avoidance of HIV transmission through sterilization of hypodermic needles. Tattooing also may increase the risk of HIV transmission in prisons (*see* "Tatooing and Body Piercing," page 9).

In addition to the appropriateness of intervention, prison officials also grapple with the time of intervention. Is the optimal time for program implementation prior to incarceration for those indicted and awaiting due process from the court system; after persons are sentenced and serving time; upon release from prison during probation or parole; or at the completion of the sentence?

According to data compiled by the Bureau of Justice Statistics, 23,404 inmates in state prisons were HIV-positive in 1995 (2.4 percent of the total population); in federal prisons, the number totaled 822 (.9 percent of the population). Of all inmates in U.S. prisons, 5,099 inmates (.5 percent) had confirmed AIDS, and 18,165 inmates were HIV-positive. In 1995, 1,010 state inmates died of AIDS-related causes, up from 955 in 1994. For every 100,000 state inmates in 1995, 100 died of AIDS-related causes. According to the Centers for Disease Control, at least 4,588 adult inmates in U.S. prisons and jails had died as a result of AIDS by the end of 1994; and during 1994, at least 5,279 adult inmates with AIDS were incarcerated in prisons and jails. At year-end 1995, 2.3 percent of all state and federal prison inmates were reported by prison authorities to be infected with the human immunodeficiency virus (HIV).

Tuberculosis

Prisons and jails are high-risk settings for the spread of TB infection. Living conditions invariably are crowded, and many facilities have extremely poor ventilation and air circulation. Moreover, many inmates already have elevated risk for TB because of their lifestyles, inadequate prior health care, and increased prevalence of HIV/AIDS. A recent study of the New York City jail system demonstrates that TB infection and progression to active TB disease occur at higher rates in individuals with more frequent incarceration and longer total time spent in jail.

Tuberculosis is not a new problem in prisons and jails. Several studies undertaken in correctional facilities in New York City, New Orleans, and Arkansas between the mid-1940s and the late 1970s revealed higher rates of TB infection and disease among inmates than in the outside population. Several of these studies also documented the transmission of TB infection among inmates and from recently released offenders to people in the community.

Tuberculosis is a well-recognized problem in correctional facilities nationwide. In recent years, dramatic increases in TB cases have been reported in correctional facilities in some geographic areas of the United States. Among inmates of the New York State correctional system, for example, the incidence of TB increased from 15.4 per 100,000 in 1976 and 1978, to 105.5 per 100,000 in 1986. In 1994, the number of TB cases among residents of correctional facilities for 59 reporting areas had reached 24,361 (4.6 percent of the total reporting correctional population).

By 1993, this incidence rate was 139.3 per 100,000. In addition, the unadjusted case rates for prison populations in many areas are markedly higher than the rates for the general population. The 1993 TB case rate of 139.3 per 100,000 in the New York State correctional system was more than six times the case rate of 21.7 per 100,000 for the general population of New York State. Similarly, in New Jersey, the incidence of TB among state inmates in 1992 was 91.3 per 100,000, compared with 12.6 per 100,000 for the state's general population in the same year. At one California state prison, the annual incidence rate of TB in 1991 was 184 cases per 100,000, more than ten times the statewide annual incidence rate. Transmission of TB also was documented in this California prison.

In several recent TB outbreaks in correctional facilities, failure to detect active TB disease in inmates resulted in transmission of TB to other inmates, correctional facility employees, and people in the community. Moreover, outbreaks in New York and California have involved the transmission of multi drug-resistant strains of TB to both inmates and employees of correctional facilities.

Call to Action

There is an enormous personal, familial, and public health price to pay for treatment intervention after the onset of HIV/AIDS, sexually transmitted diseases, and TB. This realization may account for the considerable increase in attention and support for prevention programs directed toward reducing the damage manifested in our society by risky sexual behavior, illicit drug use, and population density. Correctional administrators must confront the challenges involved in designing and deploying effective prevention strategies to confront crowding, self-destructive drug use, and sexual behaviors among prison and jail inmates. In any effective prevention program, there is a need for the target population to define the problem and participate in the assessment phase prior to implementation of an intervention. In this context, prevention is taken to mean not necessarily the complete elimination of the problem but rather a significant reduction of harm. Additionally, we must monitor closely the costs and benefits that are likely to ensue. With many infectious diseases, rehabilitation is plausible; but HIV/AIDS usually involves coping, while the infected endure the debilitating and sometimes-fatal nature of the disease.

Inmates represent a marginalized population—to many, an invisible population. Once inmates are convicted and sentenced to the correctional system, their debt to society often translates into simply serving time. Again, effective prevention efforts must garner insights from the target population (the inmates) to determine what will work best. Consulting the inmate population for ideas about prevention methods and strategies may be viewed as a radical departure from standard procedures at most facilities. However, such input and probing of inmates is essential to the design of an effective prevention program.

Public health professionals should collaborate with correctional administrators to formulate and implement policies regarding HIV/AIDS, sexually transmitted diseases, and TB education and prevention programs in prisons, jails, and juvenile facilities. This will mean a new, nontraditional type of outreach for state and local health-department personnel. Such agencies generally have limited their scope of intervention to noninstitutionalized members of society. Collaboration also will mean a new role for correctional administrators who have security as their primary mission.

Much like the work done in community mental health with the deinstitutionalization of the mentally ill and the use of halfway houses and other transitional facilities, public health professionals need to work with community-based organizations to facilitate the continuum of reinforcement of HIV/AIDS, sexually transmitted diseases, and TB education and prevention activities. This means that local and state public health assistance will be required by group homes, prerelease centers, and other transitional housing facilities to buttress the prevention message. Because there is no "magic bullet," inmates and ex-offenders will need reinforcement at every juncture until the message is conveyed that risky behaviors are life-threatening to themselves and to others. This message needs to be accompanied by other support systems that assist this population with counseling, testing, offering comprehensive and credible programs of interactive education, notifying partners, and practicing practical risk-reduction techniques (safer sex and safer drug injection).

The challenges for public health and corrections policymakers to address the threat of communicable diseases adequately will require deliberation and established policies on screening and testing protocols, compassionate release, isolation procedures for TB, and harm-reduction procedures (related to availability of condoms and sterile syringes). Proactive health education and prevention programs with emphasis on peer education warrants concerted attention by program planners. Moreover, collaboration with community agencies and health departments also will reduce the public health threat to the community.

References

Abeles, H. et al. 1970. The Large City Prison: A Reservoir of Tuberculosis. *American Review of Respiratory Diseases.*

American Correctional Association. 1998. "Health Care," in *Best Practices: Excellence in Corrections.* Lanham, Maryland: American Correctional Association.

Bellin, E. Y., D. D. Fletcher, and S. M. Safyer. 1993. Association of Tuberculosis Infection with Increased Time in or Admission to the New York City Jail System. *Journal of the American Medical Association.*

Braun, M. M., B. I. Truman, B. Maguire, et al. 1989. Increasing Incidence of Tuberculosis in a Prison Inmate Population: Association with HIV Infection. *Journal of the American Medical Association.*

Carrell, A. L. M. and G. J. Hart. 1990. Risk Behaviors for HIV Infection Among Drug Users in Prison. *British Medical Journal.*

Centers for Disease Control. 1992. Tuberculosis Transmission in a State Correctional Institution. California, 1990-91. *Morbidity and Mortality Weekly.*

Centers for Disease Control. 1993. Probable Transmission of Multidrug-resistant Tuberculosis in a Correctional Facility—California. *Morbidity and Mortality Weekly.*

Doll, D. C. 1988. Tattooing in Prison and HIV Infection. *Lancet.* January.

Dubler, N. N. and V. W. Sidel. 1989. On Research on HIV Infection and AIDS in Correctional Institutions. *Milbank Quarterly.*

Glaser, J. B. and R. B. Greifinger. 1993. Correctional Health Care: A Public Health Opportunity (Review). *Annals of Internal Medicine.*

Katz, J. and R. E. Plunkett. 1950. Prevalence of Clinically Significant Pulmonary Tuberculosis Among Inmates of New York State Penal Institutions. *American Review of Tuberculosis.*

King, L. and G. Geis. 1977. Tuberculosis Transmission in a Large Urban Jail. *Journal of the American Medical Association.*

Morse, D. L., B. I. Truman, J. P. Hanrahan, J. Mikl, R. K. Broaddus, B. H. Maguire, J. C. Grabau, S. Kain-Hyde, Y. Han and C. E. Lawrence. 1990. AIDS Behind Bars: Epidemiology of New York State Prison Inmate Cases, 1980-1988. *New York State Journal of Medicine.* March.

New Jersey State Department of Health, Bureau of TB Control. 1993. *Annual Report,* 1992. Trenton, New Jersey: New Jersey Department of Health.

Olivero, J. M. 1990. The Treatment of AIDS Behind the Walls of Correctional Facilities. *Social Justice.*

Room, R. 1974. Minimizing Alcohol Problems. *Alcohol, Health and Research World.* Fall.

Snider, D. E. Jr. and M. D. Hutton. 1989. Tuberculosis in Correctional Institutions. *Journal of the American Medical Association.*

Stead, W. W. 1978. Undetected Tuberculosis in Prison: Source of Infection for Community at Large. *Journal of the American Medical Association.*

Thompson, D. H. et al. 1977. Orleans Parish Prison Still Needs Program for Tuberculosis Control. *Journal of the American Medical Association.*

Valway, S. E., S. B. Richards, J. Kovacovich, R. B. Greifinger, J. T. Crawford, and S. W. Dooley. 1994. Outbreak of Multidrug-resistant Tuberculosis in a New York State Prison, 1991. *Journal of the American Medical Association.*

∾

Ronald L. Braithwaite, Ph.D., is interim chair and associate professor of the Rollins School of Public Health of Emory University. Kisha Braithwaite is a doctoral candidate at Howard University, and Ronald Poulson, Ph.D., is an assistant professor at East Carolina University.

Tattooing and Body Piercing:

Examining the Public Health Implications of These Risky Behaviors

By Ronald Braithwaite, Ph.D., Torrance Stephens, Ph.D., Nicole Bowman, M.P.H., Micah Milton, and Kisha Braithwaite

lthough tattooing is considered by some youths to be a sign of assertiveness, studies have shown that tattooing often is associated with low self-esteem, delinquency, and drug use. It is well-documented that sharing dirty syringes spreads HIV, and tattooing with dirty needles has been linked to the spread of hepatitis C, which is carried in the blood. There also is concern that tattooing, which involves putting tiny bits of ink beneath the skin, can spread HIV. With the proliferation of tattooing and body piercing, the direction of HIV intervention and prevention activities rapidly is shifting from documenting risk-reduction practices to measuring intervention outcomes.

Cause for Concern

A recent survey found that prison inmates are nearly six times more likely than the general population to have AIDS. The Centers for Disease Control and Prevention reported that 5,279 inmates had AIDS in 1994, the last year for which figures are available. This represented 5.2 cases per 1,000 inmates, while among all Americans over 18, the rate was 0.9 per 1,000. By the end of 1994, the number of AIDS deaths among inmates (during incarceration) reached 4,558.

While the number of deaths is striking, there is little research to document seroconversion during incarceration. Thus, it is not possible to say definitively that HIV has or has not been transmitted via tattooing and body piercing in prison.

Tattooing and Body Piercing

The use of illegal drugs behind bars and the use of injection drug paraphernalia is present in most U.S. prisons. Syringes that are stashed away in the prisons and used by hundreds of inmates (without knowledge of whether the "works" were bleach-cleaned) is clearly a public health threat. A 1996 survey of 4,875 Canadian inmates found that 11 percent had used illegal drugs behind bars, 45 percent had been tattooed, and 17 percent had their bodies pierced.

Tattooing and body piercing are viewed as prohibitive activities in most U.S. correctional institutions with few exceptions. Given the ban on tattooing, inmates hoard needles and ink and share contaminated equipment. Moreover, risks are exacerbated by inmates' often limited understanding of "sharing." In reality, sharing includes not only passing needles among people, but also using needles and syringes that have been used by unknown persons and perhaps not properly cleaned; sharing injection solutions (as in "backloading" and "frontloading"); and sharing containers, cotton, and other paraphernalia. When needles are not available, pieces of pens and lightbulbs sometimes are used by inmates to inject drugs, tattoo, and body pierce. Tattooing often is done with guitar strings and other expedient materials. In tattooing, sharing of the needle (or needle substitute), ink, and string used to transmit the ink may pose risks for HIV transmission.

In 1996, investigators conducted focus groups and one-on-one interviews with inmates in four correctional institutions. At one juvenile boot camp facility, they reported that tattooing was a prevalent source of possible blood contamination, and showed a higher prevalence of blood contamination than drug injection, with twelve of twenty-five inmates reporting having gotten a tattoo and only three of them having it done professionally. Nineteen knew that tattooing could transmit the AIDS virus, but it could not be determined from the survey whether this knowledge was acquired before or after the tattooing took place. Three of the inmates also reported participating in the high-risk behavior of becoming blood brothers with someone else, an old Indian ritual that involves two people cutting themselves on the hand or wrist and rubbing the cuts together.

At a detention center facility, more females (71 percent) than males (47 percent) reported having tattoos, but all of them knew that HIV could be transmitted through tattoo needles. Many reported having homemade versus professional tattoos and several reported that they had become blood brothers or sisters with someone.

A Public Health Challenge

The public health challenge posed by body piercing and tattooing in prison will require increased collaboration between correctional and public health policymakers. Such collaboration should facilitate discussions on a wide range of policy alternatives from bold harm-reduction policies to health education models using peer educators.

Since 1985, U.S. prisons and jails increasingly have incorporated HIV/AIDS education programs into their inmate orientation and prerelease activities. Nevertheless, community health officials suggest that many inmates are released carrying infectious diseases with them, hence posing a public health threat to the community at large. As a harm-reduction measure, the Correctional Service of Canada is considering allowing tattoo artists in prisons in a bid to curb the spread of disease among inmates.

The need exists for increased scientific research to document the status of tattooing and body piercing behavior in U.S. correctional facilities. Concomitantly, there is a need for more state health departments to develop regulatory mandates for tattooing and body-piercing establishments. Such policy directives could serve as guidelines for correctional systems considering harm-reduction programs related to tattooing and body piercing.

While custody and security issues are paramount, the role of protecting the health of those outside correctional facilities is associated with health education and disease-prevention programs in place in correctional facilities. After all, the vast majority of those incarcerated return to their communities after serving their sentences. Returning to communities with infectious diseases represents both a public health threat and a public health challenge.

References

Braithwaite, R., T. Hammett, and R. Mayberry. 1996. *Prisons and AIDS*. San Francisco: Jossey-Bass.

Centers for Disease Control. 1996. HIV/AIDS Education and Prevention Programs for Adults in Prisons and Jails and Juvenile Confinement Facilities. *Morbidity and Mortality Weekly*. April.

Farrow, J. A., R. H. Schwartz, and J. Vanderleeuw. 1991. Tattooing Behavior in Adolescence. *American Journal of Diseases of Children.*

Mahon, N. 1994. Let's Talk About Sex and Drugs: HIV Transmission and Prevention Behind Bars. Abstract PD 0521 presented at the 10th International Conference on AIDS, Yokohama.

Montagna, B. Personal communication, Jan. 15, 1998.

Munro, M. 1997. Tattoo Service Urged to Curb Convict Diseases. *Vancouver Sun* [online]. Available http://www.hempbc.com/cgi/me/dis/v97.n302.a14. October.

Turnbull, P. J., G. V. Stimson, and G. Stilwell. 1994. *Drug Use in Prisons.* Horsham, West Sussex, United Kingdom: AIDS Education and Research Trust.

Vidra, D. Personal communication, Jan. 15, 1998.

~

Ronald L. Braithwaite, Ph.D., is interim chair and associate professor at the Rollins School of Public Health of Emory University. Torrance Stephens, Ph.D., is a research assistant professor, and Nicole Bowman, M.P.H., and Micah Milton are research assistants at the Rollins School of Public Health of Emory University. Kisha Braithwaite is a doctoral candidate at Howard University.

Telemedicine Takes Off

Correctional Systems Across Country Embrace Cost-saving Technology

By Michelle Gailiun

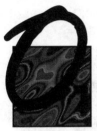n the yellowed cover of a magazine, a freckle-faced kid sits with his tongue sticking out, holding an odd-looking instrument to his chest which just might be a stethoscope. He's viewing his image on a television screen with a doctor on the other end, who looks like he may be assessing the boy's heart or lung capacity. It looks curiously like what we know of today as telemedicine. But wait a minute, the caption reads, "The Radio Doctor—Maybe," and the date is April 1924!

Telemedicine historians are fond of showing off this early cartoon from the journal *Radio News*, an uncanny representation of the modern concept of telemedicine. Clearly, someone, somewhere, was thinking way ahead. Indeed, most of the elements present in the *Radio News* cover image actually are present in one shape or another in most of today's telemedical applications.

In the broadest sense, telemedicine refers to the use of telecommunications technologies to offer health care, or clinical information, across geographic, time, or cultural barriers. Under this definition, a correctional health care worker is practicing telemedicine every time he or she picks up a telephone and talks to a physician at a local clinic about a particularly sick inmate. This definition also includes the use of faxes, store and forward computer systems, e-mail, and virtually any kind of communications technology which delivers health care or health information.

In the late 1980s, though, the term "telemedicine" was used increasingly to refer to interactive videoconferencing, in which information is exchanged through full-duplex video and audio systems, with clarity close to broadcast capability. This is the telemedicine that correctional institutions are using with increasing frequency and ease.

Modest Beginnings

Thirty years ago, the U.S. space program, the military, and many others were experimenting with the concept of remote medical care. While many of these early projects were deemed useful and successful, most folded after their grant support collapsed. A second wave of telemedicine activity was generated by another round of federal interest—and federal dollars—beginning in the late eighties and early nineties with heavy emphasis on the development of the information superhighway.

Interestingly, these developments leave state correctional institutions in a unique position to reap the benefits from years of experimentation, and to relay those lessons into practical, cost-effective telemedicine programs. Approximately three-fifths of all state correctional systems either are actively involved in telemedicine or are considering such projects, according to a recent survey by Ohio State University's Telemedicine Center.

When to Jump In

Prison populations inherently face a number of constraints which inhibit timely and adequate medical care. Many prisons are located in rural, isolated areas which are hard to reach for medical practitioners. Health care administrators often find it hard to locate and recruit enough local physicians for inmate needs. Inmates typically place high demands on the medical systems they use, and lawsuits resulting from inadequate care can cost them tens of millions of dollars. And the demands on the correctional health care system continue to grow. Nationally, prison populations are increasing at an annual rate of between 8 and 9 percent. Health care costs also continue to mount, constituting in some cases between 10 and 12 percent or even 15 percent of a state's correctional budget.

Relief is coming from several different fronts. More and more state correctional systems are privatizing part, if not all, of their medical care. Some are exploring managed-care concepts that can be transferred from a community to a correctional system, and still others are exploring telemedicine, building partnerships with major medical centers or clinics which can provide both primary and specialty care via telecommunications technologies. Telemedicine appears to be a natural fit within many correctional settings. By using sophisticated videoconferencing equipment, administrators can solve professional shortage problems by electronically connecting providers and consumers. The benefits are enormous. Security is improved because inmates do not need to travel outside their facilities for care. Travel costs are cut dramatically because the number of vans, correctional officers, and chase vehicles needed to transport inmates is reduced substantially. Through telemedicine, dozens of medical specialists are "beamed" right into a prison clinic. The same equipment electronically can "transfer" the inmate to a large urban medical center halfway across the state.

How It Works

Telemedicine usually involves two cameras, one at each site, as well as a third "document" camera for sharing important attendant data like EKGs and X-rays. The typical setup also includes one or two monitors, and in many cases, peripheral equipment like electronic stethoscopes or otoscopes which aid in diagnosis. A nurse or physician at the prison site typically presents the patient to a physician and attendant at the specialty site. Most of the time, information from the cameras, peripheral equipment, and other diagnostic tools is sent back and forth between the sites in digital format over a special phone line called a T-1 line. The best picture and motion quality come from using a full T-1 line, but since that is also the most expensive, many programs use a fraction of the line, for instance, a 1/4 T or a 1/2 T.

The equipment can be expensive, with room systems costing anywhere from $80,000 to $100,000. That cost still is less than the cost of inmate transport, however, which has been estimated to run anywhere from $100 to $800 per inmate per visit, with as many as 20,000 hospital visits per year.

Correctional systems already involved in telemedicine know that getting the equipment online is just the first step. Telemedicine requires an unusually high degree of collaboration and cooperation among various interest groups that often do not work together.

A Case Study

In a sense, Ohio is a perfect setting for telemedicine. The Ohio Department of Rehabilitation and Correction is responsible for 45,000 inmates in twenty-nine institutions, and for the last twelve years, has contracted with the Ohio State University Medical Center for specialty care. Each year, inmates make 20,000 visits to the Ohio Corrections Medical Center, about 20 minutes from the Ohio State University Medical Center. Until recently, most of the university physicians drove to the prison hospital for regularly scheduled specialty clinics. Three years ago, however, the Ohio State University Medical Center decided to implement telemedicine as a means of facilitating care, improving security, and cutting costs. It was not easy.

Under the guidance of the medical center's information systems team, the Ohio State University Medical Center and the Ohio Department of Rehabilitation and Correction chose VTEL as a vendor, and bought two double-monitored large-room systems, document cameras, and electronic stethoscopes for the two initial sites—the Corrections Medical Center and the maximum-security prison at Lucasville. But the project got off to a shaky start, as the equipment malfunctioned periodically over the first few months.

By the spring of 1995, however, the project finally began to generate regular and routine clinical care. It now boasts nine sites and may add up to six more. Physicians in eight specialties hold regular clinics and "see" approximately 200 patients per month. When the program has all sites online, the center should be able to see 300 or more patients per month.

Monitoring and evaluation procedures provide valuable feedback for participants. Site logs and continuous research reveal high patient and physician satisfaction rates. The project also is attracting grants for clinical trials in pulmonary care and community development, and administrators are beginning a pilot project within the Ohio State University Medical Center's emergency department.

Other Uses

Telemedicine systems should be easy to use, accessible, and integrated into routine systems of care delivery. The following elements are essential components of any successful telemedicine program:

- full cooperation from the highest levels of all organizations involved
- a thorough needs assessment involving all parties
- an implementation team composed of members from all organizations involved
- evaluation tools for defining and monitoring the success of the program
- a research-feedback loop

Multiple uses of the systems also enhance their value. To this end, the Ohio project, along with others, is moving to incorporate other everyday applications of videoconferencing into their systems. The Ohio State University Medical Center is offering fully accredited continuing medical education credit to the physicians at remote sites, and other plans are under way to use the system for administrative meetings and possibly parole proceedings.

Both partners in this venture see virtue in the relationship and have learned that when two parties share a vision, a third entity emerges which seems to have a life of its own—the creative energy which drives the program.

"Telemedicine is an excellent method of providing the medical services the inmates need while managing health care dollars," says Sue Devlin, a nurse who has been involved in the Ohio telemedicine project for more than a year. "The technology is expensive but will pay for itself in time and improved security."

∼

Michelle Gailiun is director of telemedicine at the Ohio State University Medical Center.

Guidelines for Implementing Inmate Medical Fees

By John Clark, M.D.

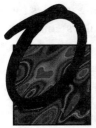

n November 9, 1994, several inmates at the Berks County Prison in Pennsylvania instituted a class action suit alleging that the prison's policy of charging inmates for medical care deprived them of their civil rights. During litigation, the plaintiffs argued that charging a fee for medical services was a barrier to medical care, and claimed that such a program severely compromised inmates' health and welfare—specifically for those with chronic diseases. The defendants argued that this was not an issue, since the Berks County Prison inmate handbook clearly articulates that services for chronic diseases which require follow-up (such as HIV, hypertension, and diabetes) are exempt.

Fortunately, the Berks County Prison's Inmate Fee for Medical Services Program had in place appropriate policies and procedures to ensure that inmates would not be denied medical care because they lacked money. When the medical records for each of the class members were reviewed, they demonstrated that policies had been followed, and that none of the class members had been denied care. Moreover, records showed that inmates with chronic medical problems had not been billed for ongoing care.

Because the Berks County Prison's Medical Services Program was well structured, with ample documentation supporting it, the court ruled in favor of the defendants. Having such a program in place is important these days, especially considering that the most frequently discussed correctional health issue during the past five years, second only to tuberculosis, has been whether or not to charge a fee for medical care provided in jails and prisons. Such discussions have intensified of late, and recent concerns have addressed many factors, including state and county funding, national health care reform, overuse of inmate medical services, jail/prison crowding, and patient responsibility in seeking health care. Regardless of the basis for implementing an inmate fee for medical care, there has been a wide range of positions on its effectiveness.

CMA/CDC

Several years ago, a focus group sponsored by the California Medical Association's Corrections and Detention Committee was charged with developing a position paper on the issue of inmate copayment for medical services. The group neither endorsed nor opposed the concept of charging inmates for health care. Members, however, did believe that decision makers could be called upon to implement "copayment" programs, regardless of personal or philosophical beliefs.

Committee members agree that, since resources are limited, it is fiscally, ethically, and politically appropriate to undertake measures which reduce waste and preserve resources. Inmates benefit through the appropriate allocation of resources, and charging a nominal fee may ensure that an inmate considers whether a health care provider's intervention is necessary. By teaching inmates to share responsibility for their own care, the committee felt that administrators may be able to enhance the value of treatment, improve its perceived effectiveness, and likely improve compliance. Furthermore, a degree of responsibility can be learned in custody and applied throughout life.

Copayment Guidelines

Despite varied opinions, inmate fee-for-medical-services programs must contain several key consensus criteria to ensure that no barriers exist which will violate the inmate's constitutional right to access medical care. The guidelines developed by the California Medical Association's Corrections and Detention Committee for the establishment of inmate copayment programs for medical services are self-explanatory. They emphasize the importance of ensuring that policies are well reasoned and clearly articulated to the inmate population. An asterisk denotes an essential criteria guideline. Guidelines are as follows:

- The program's policies and procedures must be developed jointly by custody and medical personnel.
- The fee schedule must be widely posted and/or published for inmates.*
- A list of exempt services must be published and posted.*

- A list of billable services must be published and posted.*
- A policy should be in place to waive fees for the indigent inmate.*
- A grievance/appeal process for the inmate who desires to challenge a billed service visit should be in place.*
- The copayment must be cashless.*
- A structured revenue-management system should be in place.*
- A policy should be in place to address negative balances.*
- A policy should be in place to monitor and control over-the-counter medications.
- A system should be in place to monitor morbidity and mortality annually.
- A policy should be in place to monitor the workload on the clinical service (decreases or increases in the number of clinic visits, the number of referrals to the emergency room before and after starting).
- The amount of copayment should not exceed the state rate for the Medi-Cal/Medicaid copayment.
- The program should be evaluated to ensure that it is cost effective and efficient.

Billable services would include self-initiated clinic visits, over-the-counter medications, noncrisis mental health services, and administrative fees for prescription medications (not to exceed $5 per visit). Services to be exempt would include intake medical screening, National Commission on Correctional Health Care required fourteen-day health appraisal, public health evaluations, initial mental health examinations, pregnancy-related services, services funded by special grants or contracts, laboratory and diagnostic services, life-threatening emergencies, and follow-up for chronic diseases. A list of these exempt services should be posted.

Justifying exemption is easy in many of these cases. Billing for prenatal services, for example, may place both mother and fetus at risk. Charging inmates for communicable disease screening or medical problem testing also would be inappropriate, because almost every jail and prison is under some type of state or local statute which requires officials to conduct such tests. Finally, in those cases where services are funded by special grants or contracts, billing essentially would be considered "double dipping." Case law is very clear for jails or state prisons which have billed federal inmates being housed on a per diem basis, when the per diem payment included a daily compensation for medical care.

Many individuals who are incarcerated are truly indigent and have no funds available in their inmate accounts. When applicable, there must be a mechanism to ensure that these inmates will not be denied care. In the Berks County Prison, as is the case in most institutions that bill for medical care, the service is provided first, and the decision to bill or not to bill is made after the fact, based on criteria and guidelines. In unison with the waiver process for the indigent inmate, there must be a process for an inmate to grieve or appeal a charge that has been made to his or her account.

Additionally, facility policies must be clear and specific as they relate to billable services which are provided to inmates who subsequently have funds deposited into their accounts. Policies also should address the reincarceration of an inmate who has a negative balance on the books (within a specified period of time).

Conclusion

In the Berks County Inmate Fee for Medical Services Program, all of the California Medical Association's Corrections and Detention Committee guidelines had been met, with the exception of an overall evaluation of the cost effectiveness of the program. At the time of trial in this case (May 1996), a detailed analysis of the Berks County program was discussed. In the decision rendered on August 14, 1996, the court ruled that fees for medical services programs do not per se violate the Eighth and Fourteenth Amendments of the U.S. Constitution for sentenced inmates and pretrial detainees. The court recommended that notices and literature about the program be published in English and Spanish to ensure that information was conveyed effectively to non-English-speaking inmates.

In terms of the growing body of experience with fee-for-medical-services programs, the number of clinic/sick call visits generally has decreased in the first months following implementation of the new program, and has returned to preprogram statistics in about one year. As outlined in the California Medical Association's Corrections and Detention Committee criteria, it is extremely important to have an objective evaluation of these programs in place to ensure that they are meeting the stated goals and objectives of the agency.

The goal of reducing unnecessary visits to "Sick Call" is an inappropriate reason to start such an inmate fee-for-medical-services program, regardless of the reason or number of times a client seeks the services of medical staff. Each visit should be viewed as an opportunity to evaluate a high-risk population for the presence of clinically significant pathologies.

As a consultant and expert witness on many cases involving inmate deaths, this author has reviewed a number of cases where patients were not objectively evaluated for a specific complaint because they had acquired the label of a "malingerer." These inmates invariably succumb to premature death, which has resulted in avoidable and unnecessary liability for correctional facilities.

~

Dr. John Clark has been chief medical officer for the Los Angeles County Sheriff's Office for the past eleven years.

Mental Illness as a Chronic Condition:

Coping with Chronic Mental Patients in a Correctional Setting

By Robert S. Ort, M.D., Ph.D. and
Kenneth L. Faiver, M.P.H.

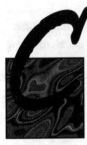orrectional officials used to have a saying: "Most inmates are bad, but some are sad and a few are mad." It meant that most inmates were truly obnoxious characters, but some of them were depressed, and a few were so obviously mentally ill as to require professional mental health treatment.

The Diagnostic and Statistical Manual of Mental Disorders (DSM-IV)—the major reference manual for mental health professionals—catalogs and defines almost every conceivable mental disorder. Comprised of hundreds of pages, it contains substantially more diagnostic categories than "bad, sad or mad." It also describes the various factors that mental health professionals must consider before reaching a diagnosis and preparing a long-term treatment plan.

Our society generally disapproves of the punishment of mentally ill people for behavior resulting from impaired understanding and control. But it happens all the time. Too few community resources are available to permit adequate and timely response to concerns raised about behaviors of mentally ill people—many of whom also are homeless and/or on drugs. Police find themselves with insufficient alternatives in these circumstances, so the mentally ill are arrested and held in jail on a variety of charges. The unfortunate consequences are well known.

Now that sheriffs, jail administrators, and prison wardens are responsible for operating facilities which contain large numbers of mentally ill individuals, some of the traditional methods of managing inmates may be outmoded. The more effective and humane management of mentally ill inmates may require a radically different approach.

Society's Failure

One hundred and fifty years ago, jails and almshouses were becoming repositories of the mentally ill. Beginning in the 1840s, Dorothea Dix, Horace Mann, and others labored long and hard to change this situation and placed strong emphasis on establishing state and county psychiatric hospitals. By 1880, more than 75 such hospitals were in existence, while less than 1 percent of inmates in jails and prisons were reported to have serious mental illness. From about 1880 to the end of World War II, states were viewed as meeting their ethical and moral obligations if they provided hospital care to patients with acute mental illness and humane custodial care to those with chronic mental illness. However, during the 1930s and 1940s, periodic media reports described deplorable conditions in these hospitals, including physical neglect, sexual abuse, and inhumane treatment. The resulting outcries set the stage for deinstitutionalization. After World War II, a sustained attack on the legitimacy of mental hospitalization emerged.

The Kennedy administration initiated its "bold new approach" to treatment of the mentally ill in 1963, with the promise of 2,000 community mental health centers—enabling a shift from costly institutional care to what was touted as more cost-effective and humane care in the community. During the Carter administration, there was a resurgence of support for continued deinstitutionalization, along with incorporation of the principle that patients with severe mental illness should be treated in the least-restrictive setting. The inertia of deinstitutionalization persists to this day. Some states are at the point of discharging the last few hundred mentally ill patients from their remaining institutions.

To appreciate the full thrust of this phenomenon, a clear understanding of its definition is necessary. Deinstitutionalization is a process with two components: (1) the transfer of people from their institutional environments to the community, and (2) the prevention of hospitalization for those people who might be considered potential candidates for hospital care.

Deinstitutionalization, since 1978, has been based on the principle that severe mental illness should be treated in the least-restrictive setting. This laudable goal has been realized at least partially for many. But for a substantial minority, it is a dismal failure. These are the people who are unable to adapt to living with their families, in group homes, or in flophouses. They are the people who now sleep in doorways, under bridges, in cardboard boxes, or in our prison and jail cells.

This last phenomenon has been called the "criminalization of the mentally ill." It is estimated that as many as 10 to 15 percent of inmates in prisons and jails are seriously mentally ill and in need of psychiatric care, and that up to 5 percent are actively psychotic, that is, actively responding to their delusions and hallucinations. Jail officials in Wayne County, Michigan, which includes Detroit, report that nearly 17 percent of jail inmates are taking psychotropic medication. Since 1993, the number of Michigan inmates who were previously in state mental hospitals has grown at twice the rate of the general prison population. These patients require treatment similar to what they received or would receive in the free world.

Antitherapeutic Nature Of Incarceration

The health records of mentally ill inmates typically contain notes written by psychiatrists, social workers, psychologists, and nurses addressing such topics as mental status, suicidal ideation, response to medication, and current symptoms. However, only rarely do they document the history of mental illness and the patient's prior treatment experience. Even less often do prison health professionals inquire about adjustment to current surroundings or about important events that are occurring in their patients' lives, such as their trials, sentencing, prospects of prison, appeals, visitors (or lack thereof), well-being of children, or unfaithfulness or abandonment by spouse or significant other.

Nevertheless, each of these can be significant—even momentous—events or concerns for the confined person. Consistent failure to explore these aspects of the patients' lives suggests that mental health staff already may have accepted the antitherapeutic environment of a prison or jail as an unchangeable reality. In abdicating the role of change agent, the professional becomes less effective therapeutically. It is inexcusable for mental health staff to ignore the major stress factors affecting patients, since the presence of such factors may indicate specific treatment modifications.

Confinement itself is highly stressful. A jail or prison is not a very comforting, reassuring, or stabilizing environment—even in the best of circumstances.

Mental Illness as a Chronic Condition

As psychiatrist E. Fuller Torrey comments, "Being in jail or prison when your brain is working normally is, at best, an unpleasant experience. Being in jail or prison when your brain is playing tricks on you is often brutal."

In prison, the inmate is exposed to frequent loud noises. He or she must associate with predatory and dangerous people. He or she lives in constant fear and uncertainty, not knowing whom to trust. The environment is strange and unfamiliar. There is little opportunity to exercise meaningful control over one's life. In addition, jail inmates may experience considerable anxiety over their trial and sentencing or over recent separation from loved ones.

Second only to medication, the environment (milieu) in which a person lives is the single most powerful factor influencing the course of illness, the efficacy of treatment interventions, and the patient's response to external stimuli. The nature of the environment has a direct bearing on how quickly a patient will decompensate, how severe the episode will become, and how stable the patient will be (course of illness). A beneficial change in the efficacy of treatment interventions may result from a nurturing and supportive environment that encourages compliance with medication; however, the benefits of treatment can be eroded or negated by stressful surroundings.

Finally, while a person may respond appropriately to stressful stimuli taken one at a time, it may be impossible to cope when the whole environment is stressful. Crowding has been known to exacerbate the stresses of institutional life and compound the endemic problems of prisons and jails, including poor living conditions, lack of meaningful work, interinmate violence, sexual exploitation, and weakening of the inmate's usual affectional ties.

However, for some mentally ill inmates, the correctional environment can offer a positive improvement over what was experienced on the outside. At least, they have food, clothing, and shelter, as well as access to medical and dental care, mental health treatment, counseling, and rehabilitative programming. It is only because of the extremely deprived and hostile environments from which these people come that the correctional setting can be regarded as relatively less stressful.

A Chronic Condition

Jails and prisons have become, by default, the public institutions for care of the mentally ill in our society. Jail and prison personnel no longer can say that mentally ill inmates belong in state hospitals. For practical purposes, there are no state mental hospitals. As a consequence, jails and prisons must establish treatment programs for mentally ill inmates. Such programs should provide for the safety, security, and humane treatment of this segment of the incarcerated population.

To establish an effective program for the care and treatment of seriously mentally ill inmates, one must understand the nature, composition, and size of this group. The first, and perhaps the largest, subgroup comprises deinstitutionalized patients who are older and have histories of multiple hospitalizations. Younger patients, on the other hand, usually do not have a history of multiple admissions to state hospitals because there have been no beds for them. Both groups of patients, the young and the old, over time will be diagnosed as demonstrating symptoms of severe mental illness, for example, schizophrenia, bipolar disorder, major depression, or psychoses.

The mental illness typically found in these groups of patients is chronic in nature. Chronic mental illness, unlike many physical conditions, is not cured by treatment. Pneumonia, for instance, is cured by a single dose of penicillin. A fractured forearm, properly aligned and cast, will mend in about six weeks. But with an illness like arthritis, acute symptoms (pain and stiffness) quickly return once treatment is discontinued or when the patient experiences stressful conditions such as cold or extreme changes in barometric pressure. The same is true of such mental conditions as schizophrenia, bipolar disorder, major depression, and other psychoses.

Twenty years ago, when much less was known about how the brain functions, it was considerably easier to speculate about the underlying causes of mental illness. Now, with the advances in our knowledge about the biochemistry, neuropathways, and anatomy of the brains of chronically mentally ill people, in comparison to the brains of normal people, the field is notably more complex. We know, for instance, that the concentration of certain chemicals in normal brains differs from that found in the brains of chronically mentally ill patients. Second, we know from studies of identical twins that the ventricles in the brain of a schizophrenic twin are larger than those of the twin who is normal. Third, it has been amply demonstrated that mentally ill people employ different portions of their brains than do normal people when performing the same intellectual functions, giving evidence of a physiological rationale for their less effective coping skills.

We know also that an illness such as the flu can initiate a bout of depression in chronically mentally ill patients. We know that for patients with chronic mental illness, medication is the primary treatment. We know that the second most effective treatment for these patients is placement in a therapeutic environment. In such a setting, members of the treatment team can aid the patient by helping to establish or reestablish contact with significant others, or by offering reassurance, clarification, and comfort, when needed.

A patient treated with medication in a therapeutic environment often reaches a state of remission in which the more flagrant symptoms have subsided. Because of the chronic nature of mental illness, the treatment plan must address long-term care and treatment even after the patient has been stabilized on medication and no longer requires the intensive services of a hospital or other acute care setting. Although medication protects against relapse, helps to maintain stability, and assists a mentally ill person in coping with life's stresses, it cannot fully protect against more extreme forms of stress, especially when combined with limited problem-solving skills or loss of social support. This helps to explain why, even with medication, about 40 percent of newly discharged schizophrenic patients in the free world tend to relapse within a year of their discharge from a hospital. In fact, psychosocial treatment is most helpful for patients who are not exhibiting severe psychotic symptoms and who have reached a degree of stability through faithful compliance with their medication.

Looking at chronic mental illness in these terms, only a few mentally ill inmates can be discharged from a mental health unit into the general population of a jail or prison and be expected to make an adequate adjustment. Consequently, there should be a plan for ongoing care of a large proportion of the mentally ill population. This plan should involve housing that is designed to afford relief from the typical sources of stress found in the general population. Correctional administrators who do not have such a plan risk falling into the deinstitutionalization trap once again—this time within their own facilities.

Some inmates exhibit signs of mental illness for the first time shortly after being exposed to extreme levels of stress in a jail or prison. Similar episodes of disabling anxiety, psychosis, depression, agitation, or mania—often referred to as "shell shock"—also were reported in both world wars. Typically, treatment of this initial episode will result in a subsiding of the symptoms, at which point the inmate can be returned to the general population because a repeat episode is highly unlikely.

Two chronic mental illnesses that often are not diagnosed in correctional facilities are post-traumatic stress disorder and the psychiatric disorders associated with severe head trauma. Yet, an appreciable number of inmates suffer from such conditions. If, for example, the clinician were to arrive at a clinical association between head trauma and explosive episodes, it might lead to a relevant treatment strategy rather than a punishing response to the patient's behavior. The therapist might learn through interviews with the patient, correctional officers, and family members that he had led a normal life up to the age of ten when he was hit in the head with a baseball bat, after which he was hospitalized and did not regain consciousness for four days. Subsequently, he responded inappropriately—and often violently—to frustrating circumstances. From his history, the therapist reasonably might conclude that there is a connection between the head injury and the patient's abrupt change in behavior, and that mental health treatment is likely to be a more effective answer than time spent in disciplinary segregation.

Mental Health Units

Even well-managed correctional environments can be inherently hostile to the mentally ill because of the characteristic noise, crowding, fears, separation from loved ones, abuse, and threats from predatory inmates, lack of normal amenities, idleness, anxiety over trial and sentencing, shame, embarrassment, and loss of hope. Several of these factors in combination can be extremely stressful and may push a person "over the edge." An otherwise stable person may become acutely mentally ill under these circumstances. Some are stabilized readily with medication. Others need only a brief assist from supportive therapists. But many do not get along well in the general correctional environment. Without daily encouragement, they fail to take their medications regularly. They begin to hear and respond to voices and other internal stimuli, and become overly fearful and paranoid. They behave in bizarre, offensive, and injurious ways.

Mental Illness as a Chronic Condition

An increasing number of correctional systems have found it useful to establish inpatient units and intermediate care settings for mentally ill inmates who, from time to time, experience severe symptoms. But often, the number of beds in these units is inadequate, given the high percentage of mentally ill inmates. Correctional authorities and mental health professionals sometimes find it necessary to adopt a strategy of discharging the less severely ill to the general population in order to make room for the more severely ill. When fragile and unstable patients are discharged to the general population, the combination of environmental stressors and poor medication compliance contribute quickly to an increase in symptoms. These patients then are returned to the mental health unit—but not before experiencing severe pain and distress, and possibly having even injured themselves or others.

The establishment of therapeutic environments within correctional facilities affords greater opportunity for staff to observe and monitor patients for timely indications of change in behavior or mental status, thus providing an early warning before adverse behavior erupts. The daily reminders from nursing staff and the example of peers tend to encourage compliance with prescribed treatment. Patients feel safer; indeed, they are safer from harm from themselves or others. Many of the disturbing stimuli characteristic of the general population setting have been eliminated or minimized. Staff take the time to encourage adequate nutritional intake, good sleep habits, and proper hygiene and grooming. Through frequent and ready access to care staff, patients develop a "therapeutic alliance" with caregivers, which fosters participation in treatment activities and ensures that patients receive reassurance and support in the face of troubling internal stimuli or adverse external events. Finally, patients in such a unit have greatly improved access to regular professional evaluation and treatment.

But separate mental health units also serve an additional purpose. Mentally ill inmates can disrupt entire housing units. Some inmates take delight in baiting or abusing the mentally impaired. Others feel annoyance at their behavior and tend to behave in inappropriate ways. The general population of the institution is demonstrably quieter and more manageable once the mentally ill are moved to another setting.

Classification

Mentally ill inmates who are appropriately classified at each treatment level have certain common characteristics. These treatment levels go by various names, such as intensive care, acute care, active care, subacute care, intermediate care, residential care, and outpatient care. See Figure 1 on page 34 for the typical characteristics of patients requiring these levels of care.

In the community, lengths of stay in acute psychiatric hospitals have become quite short, and the mentally ill tend to remain longer in community care settings (residential treatment centers). But one should be wary of applying the community mental health guidelines to inmates without making appropriate adjustments. For many, the stresses experienced behind bars are immeasurably more severe than those they have encountered in the free world. Without extra help and support, people who perhaps could do well at home with a caring family member are unable to cope adequately in the jail or prison setting. Moreover, commonly accepted intervals for follow-up of chronic patients in the community make an assumption that a given patient is known to be sufficiently stable to tolerate thirty-day, ninety-day, or longer periods without follow-up.

Until the patient's response pattern in the correctional environment is observed fully and evaluated, much more frequent contact is needed. Likewise, when a patient is moved from a higher to a lower intensity of care, therapeutic contact should be frequent until the patient is stable, and only then should it be decreased gradually.

Failure to See Chronic Nature of Mental Illness

Recognizing that mental illness is a chronic condition has significant policy implications. Some of the practices commonly seen in correctional systems can be attributed to a misunderstanding in this area. Mental health professionals working in correctional settings have a responsibility to raise these issues whenever, in their professional judgment, the health and well-being of patients are affected adversely.

Mentally ill inmates who are treated in a hospital or mental health unit may be returned too quickly to the general population. The environment of the mental health unit is safe, comforting, and structured. Staff are supportive.

Figure 1

Typical Characteristics of Patients Requiring Active Level of Care
Suicidal
Homicidal
Severely disturbed
Highly unstable
Agitated
Severe psychiatric/neuropsychiatric symptoms
Experiencing treatment complications
Persistent diagnostic uncertainty
Severe personal distress/psychic pain
Unable to cope with demands of everyday life within the jail or prison
Requires major assistance with activities of daily living
Requires titration of various psychoactive medications
Acute psychoactice substance withdrawal
Severe or persistent self-mutilative behavior

Typical Characteristics of Patients Requiring Subacute Care
Superficial self-injurious behavior
Moderate agitation, psychotic symptoms, psychic pain, psychiatric distress
Requires some assistance with activities of daily living

Typical Characteristics of Patients Requiring Residential Care
Patient likely to decompensate in general population
Low level of psychic distress
History of chronic mental illness
No suicidal or homicidal intent
Chronic illness is stable
Unable to cope with demands of everyday life within the jail or prison
Able to care for personal activities of daily living and grooming with minimal
    assistance and encouragement
Symptoms are no longer extreme
Patient's symptoms and behaviors frequently provoke disciplinary sanctions
Definitive diagnosis has been made
Vulnerability to victimization

Typical Characteristics of Patients Requiring Outpatient Care
No history of mental illness, single episode of psychiatric disorder
History of long remissions when kept on medication
History of dependable compliance with medication regimen
Patients recompensate with little or no pharmacotherapy
Behaviors are not overly offensive or provocative to other inmates

---

Disturbing and hostile stimuli are absent or minimized. Patients are encouraged to take their medication regularly. But upon arrival in the general population, they are subjected to insults and threats from other inmates, unpleasant sights and noise, indignities and discomforts, and little or no encouragement to take their medication regularly. Not surprisingly, their symptoms recur. Professional staff should not be too quick to say that a patient is stabilized and can return to the general population. It is all right to try a person out in the general population, but a long-term assignment to a sheltered living unit should be considered if the placement is not successful.

Failure to appreciate the chronicity of mental illness leads to substitution of crisis intervention for regular follow-up care. The treatment plan for patients discharged from a mental health unit should specify a regular program of therapeutic contact, rather than reliance on crisis intervention. Case management strategies for general population inmates can be helpful in ensuring continuity of care.

Treatment staff should be attentive to sources of stress in the patient's daily life. As already indicated, one such significant source, in a jail, is the course of the trial and sentencing. Another area of concern to mental health staff is placement of a mental patient in segregation, and this for two reasons: the events that led to segregation may be indicative of a developing problem, and the circumstances of the segregation environment are likely to be stressful and may provoke further symptoms.

It is said frequently that a mental health unit should be made uncomfortable so as to discourage malingering. This advice deserves careful reevaluation. Does it really make sense to deliberately create an unpleasant, antitherapeutic environment for a mental health unit? Do we seriously want to reduce the overall effectiveness of a treatment program just to discourage possible overutilization? It is best to entrust skilled clinicians with the task of determining who needs to be admitted and who should be discharged. It is better to allow a few unnecessary days in the unit by an occasional inappropriate patient than to render the entire program less than optimally effective. Also, inmates who quickly develop severe symptoms upon return to the general population should not be rashly labeled malingerers who just want to enjoy the comfortable mental health unit. Normal people do not often seek the constant company of mental patients for "enjoyment and comfort." On the other hand, the truly mentally ill person is especially vulnerable to stressful situations.

All too often, standard correctional practices of punishment are inflicted on inmates known to be mentally ill. If the mentally ill patient is in a treatment program, untoward behavior is best dealt with in a therapeutic manner. Punitive methods rarely have been found to help control the disruptive behavior of mental patients. The treatment team should employ clinically appropriate strategies in response to difficult and refractory behavior.

∼

Robert S. Ort, M.D., Ph.D., is a psychiatrist and clinical psychologist who served eight years as director of psychiatry for the Michigan Department of Corrections. Kenneth L. Faiver, M.P.H., managed the health program for the Michigan Department of Corrections for sixteen years and then served three years as chief medical coordinator for the correctional system of Puerto Rico. He now is president of Correctional Health Resources Inc. and is the author of Health Care Management Issues in Corrections, *published by the American Correctional Association.*

References

Deutsch, Albert. 1948. *The Shame of the States*. New York: Harcourt Brace.

Faiver, K. 1998. *Health Care Management Issues in Corrections*. Lanham, Maryland: American Correctional Association.

Hornbeck, Mark. 1997. Mentally Ill Flood Prisons. *The Detroit News*. (Page 13A).

Roth, Loren H. 1968. Correctional Psychiatry. In William J. Curran, A. Louis McGarry, and Saleem A. Shah, eds. *Forensic Psychiatry and Psychology*. Philadelphia, Pennsylvania: F. A. Davis Company.

Torrey, E. Fuller, 1997. *Out of the Shadows: Confronting America's Mental Illness Crisis*. New York: John Wiley & Sons Inc.

Staff Health and Wellness:

Protecting the Health of Correctional Employees Is a Long-Term Endeavor

By Lester N. Wright, M.D., M.P.H.

The deaths of several inmates and a correctional officer from multiple drug-resistant tuberculosis in 1991 convinced the New York State Department of Correctional Services to implement significant changes in its health programs, not only for inmates but also for its employees. The Department of Correctional Services' response was to create a unit of communicable disease consultant nurses within its Health Services Division; this provided the staffing required to greatly strengthen its disease prevention programs. In the last six years, the Department of Correctional Services' approach to health protection has become much more systematized, and the numbers have reflected this improvement.

As the Department of Correctional Services moves toward the year 2000, under the leadership of Governor George E. Pataki and Corrections Commissioner Glenn S. Goord, it continues to advance its commitment to protect the health, well-being, and safety of the 31,000 employees in its sixty-nine American Correctional Association-accredited facilities. There are five elements comprising this commitment: education and training; employee assistance programs; monitoring and surveillance; health services; and clear directives, policies, and planning. These elements are supported and implemented by both state- and facility-level administrators, employee unions, and various committees working together to create a climate that promotes health and safety for all.

Wellness Training

Employee awareness of health and safety issues within the Department of Correctional Services begins during initial training at the Albany Training Academy. As correctional officers learn how to function safely and effectively in a prison culture, they also learn how to improve their chances of staying healthy in the midst of a relatively unhealthy population. Similarly, these topics are part of the facility orientation program that nonuniformed employees receive. For both, the health-protection emphasis continues on an annual basis. Mandatory annual employee health and safety education and training is provided in each facility. Tuberculosis education; protection from blood-borne pathogens, including HIV and hepatitis B; and personal protective equipment are among the mandated courses. In addition, fire and safety training covers fire prevention techniques, the use of fire emergency equipment and evacuation procedures, as well as prevention of accidents and injury.

Right-to-know training focuses on the law pertaining to the promotion of a healthy environment and includes Occupational Safety and Health Administration (OSHA) requirements and the New York State Hazard Communication Standards. Chemical agents training reviews safety issues and correct use of chemical agents within the correctional setting. Stress II training provides informative insights into hostage situations should they occur within the department. All of these courses are part of each employee's forty annual training hours required by the American Correctional Association accreditation standards.

An Employee Assistance Program (EAP) has been established in each correctional facility. This program serves correctional employees and/or their families, and also is available to retirees. Under the guidance of a local labor management committee, each facility provides employees with access to a variety of community programs, including medical and mental health assessments, counseling, and support groups.

Tracking Disease

The Health Services Division's Communicable and Infectious Disease Unit monitors both inmates and staff for acute infectious diseases. This unit implements systems to evaluate, diagnose, treat, and follow up cases of infectious disease. The unit also promotes educational initiatives designed to emphasize prevention. Infection control nurses work as consultants to facility staff and promote communication and cooperation between groups concerned with these issues both inside and outside the Health Services Division. The Department of Correctional Services works closely with the New York State Department of Health, county, and local health departments, hospitals, and other correctional jurisdictions to arrange for continuity of care for both employees and inmates.

The Department of Correctional Services mandates and provides annual PPD (tuberculosis) testing for everyone in the system, including inmates, employees, and volunteers. Since 1993, the rate of TB skin test conversions (which indicate transmission of new infection) of staff has decreased from 1.7 percent to .2 percent as the Department of Correctional Services has implemented a policy which requires not only mandatory annual testing but also liberal use of negative-pressure isolation rooms, directly observed administration of all TB medications, and extensive contact investigations. The education that staff and inmates receive about TB enables everyone in the system to recognize symptoms that may result from TB and refer anyone with symptoms for evaluation.

The Department of Correctional Services also provides hepatitis B immunization for any of its staff who may come in contact with blood. These usually are begun during initial training for correctional officers and continued according to the standard immunization schedule. This provides a high degree of protection against hepatitis B for employees.

HIV/AIDS Prevention

The Department of Correctional Services has been involved heavily in treating and preventing transmission of human immunodeficiency virus (HIV) since the disease was first recognized in the early 1980s. Although the rate of HIV infection in males entering the system has continued to decrease for the last several years and now stands at 7 percent, the rate among incoming females has increased to 18 percent. Factoring in length of stay, the Department of Correctional Services estimates it currently has custody of 7,500 HIV-positive inmates. Thus, staff exposure to HIV (and to hepatitis B) has been a major concern. All employees receive annual training about blood-borne diseases, emphasizing the use of universal precautions to protect against blood exposure. Engineering solutions such as the wide availability of latex gloves, the use of safety injection needles, and the training of staff and inmate crews in the cleanup of blood spills can minimize but not eliminate risk.

When the Centers for Disease Control and Prevention published recommendations on post-exposure prophylaxis in mid-1996, the Department of Correctional Services studied them and tried to determine how to implement them in its far-flung system. The Centers for Disease Control guidelines recommend that prophylaxis after significant exposure begin within one-to-two hours. But, as in many states, some of New York's correctional facilities are located in rural areas where access to specialist medical care is difficult. What if the exposure occurs at 2 A.M. in a facility that is miles from the nearest medical center or even from the nearest pharmacy? After explaining the situation to its employee unions and obtaining approval from the state boards of nursing and pharmacy, the Department of Correctional Services established stock kits containing seventy-two-hour supplies of the required medications that can be made available to exposed employees until they are able to obtain care from their private providers. These stock kits are available in all facilities.

Blood Emergency Response Teams (BERT) are volunteer services operated jointly by the Department of Correctional Services and its employee unions that provide support to employees who may have experienced a significant blood exposure. Their services are confidential and are offered upon employee request. BERT members are trained correctional employee volunteers. Their mission is to assist employees with knowledge, support, and guidance in addition to that provided by the health services staff. Their service also is extended to the employee's family, when requested.

Employees' health records and computerized data travel with them to other state correctional facilities upon transfer. This enables employees to have an updated employee health history at all times.

Policies and Planning

Up-to-date and clear directives, policies, and planning are the backbone of employee health, well-being, and safety. The New York Department of Correctional Services maintains directives on TB contact investigations, the TB control program, and respiratory protection. Health service policies include an employee HIV/hepatitis B postexposure protocol and tuberculosis control. These directives and policies are reviewed annually to keep the department consistent with current health practices.

A Health and Safety Committee that includes members from health services, labor relations, facilities planning, and the three bargaining units (which represent the Department of Correctional Services' employees) addresses employee health and safety issues on a regular basis. Inclusion of facilities planning staff in the discussions ensures that health units comply with ever-changing codes and regulations. These have required extensive updating of older facilities, as well as extensive health facility construction projects.

Many facilities are located in older buildings, some of which are more than 150 years old. Although they have been remodeled repeatedly since originally constructed, some health services units resemble museums. The Department of Correctional Services recognized that it was much harder to protect employee health and safety, and provide services efficiently, in outdated buildings, and made a major commitment to a "Health Care Plan of Action" to update or replace those units. Planning and constructing enough modern health care units to provide for delivery of the large volume of health care services needed by its inmates is an ongoing, multiyear project.

No matter what an employee's job responsibilities may be, he or she is entitled to work in a safe and healthy environment. The key to meeting the staff health and wellness needs of each employee is to implement an employee wellness plan that protects against known risks and is adaptable to meet future ones. The five elements described here—education and training; employee assistance programs; monitoring and surveillance; health services; and clear directives, policies, and planning—form the cornerstone of any employee wellness program. The Department of Correctional Services recognizes that it takes hundreds of hands working together to make it happen.

≈

Lester N. Wright, M.D., M.P.H., is the associate commissioner and chief medical officer for the New York State Department of Correctional Services.

Meeting the Challenges of Juvenile Health Care

By James Farrow, M.D.

*T*he health care needs and status of incarcerated youths have received limited public policy and programmatic attention. But with the rising number of children and adolescents involved in both the adult and juvenile justice systems, their health problems and level of health services needed have become more pressing in recent years.

Although adolescence generally is a time of vigorous health, the health problems that do occur among teenagers often go untreated. Poor health frequently results from risky behavior or emotional distress. Inexperience with adult roles and behaviors, coupled with changes in thinking processes, may lead adolescents to make poor judgments and behave unwisely, leading to pregnancy, sexually transmitted diseases, or motor vehicle accidents related to the use of alcohol or drugs. Adolescence also is a period when serious mental health problems may be identified, including severe anxiety, depression, and suicidal thoughts.

Correctional administrators not only should be aware of the myriad health problems affecting incarcerated youths, but should work with local and state health departments to provide those services most needed to improve the quality of care for incarcerated children and adolescents.

Prevalence of Disease

For a variety of reasons, research has shown that youths who enter the juvenile justice system or any other correctional system are more likely than their peers to suffer from health problems. Medical problems were diagnosed in

46 percent of 47,000 adolescents in a New York City youth detention facility over an 11-year period. Dental problems were diagnosed in 90 percent of these adolescents. In a 1979 investigation conducted by the American Medical Association, incarcerated youths had higher-than-average rates of many health problems, including seizure disorders; respiratory illness; obesity and other nutritional disorders; bone and joint problems; skin ailments; and dental disease. Similar findings have been reported in a number of more recent studies with offenders in short-term detention facilities.

Studies focused on human immunodeficiency virus (HIV) seropositivity among incarcerated juveniles reveal infection rates ranging from less than 1 percent to close to 20 percent. Differences in infection rates may be explained in part by regional variations in transmission rates, regional substance abuse patterns, and the ethnicity of the populations involved. In one investigation of behavioral risks for HIV infection, incarcerated youths reported several risk factors, including having three or more sexual partners (35.6 percent), engaging in homosexual behavior (2 percent), having anal sex (19 percent), and having sex with an intravenous drug user (14.4 percent). A number of studies of youthful offenders have found that the majority of detainees in both short- and long-term facilities have used cigarettes, alcohol, and illicit substances. Many detainees had been sexually victimized.

Confined youthful offenders are much more likely to be from poor families, who have provided inadequate health care and supervision. Confinement may exacerbate pre-existing health problems or contribute to new ones. For example, juveniles may suffer injuries as a result of fights, assaults, or self-mutilation. Staff attempts to control youthful detainees through use of handcuffs, other restraints, or excessive medication also can lead to health problems.

In addition to their physical health problems, a large proportion of incarcerated youths have significant mental health problems. Research and clinical experience suggest a higher incidence of mental illness, emotional disturbance, mental retardation, and other developmental disabilities among confined juveniles than among those in the general population. In addition, several studies of incarcerated youths indicate that they frequently suffer from major depression and report an unusually high rate of suicide attempts. Learning disabilities, Attention Deficit Hyperactivity Disorder, and other behavioral and conduct disorders also appear to be significantly more prevalent among incarcerated youths. Many facilities that confine juveniles have responded to this increased health need by developing special mental health units or enhancing mental health services for the entire inmate population.

Health Services

The health care problems of incarcerated youths demonstrate the need for a comprehensive system of health care delivery within correctional facilities. Ideally, this system of care should be coordinated by an adolescent health care professional and should include assessment, diagnosis, and treatment. Nationwide, there are many variations in the systems of health care delivery for incarcerated juvenile populations, but the care generally falls into three categories: 1) an on-site, comprehensive care model involving a complete medical and mental health team of physicians and nurses; 2) an on-site, limited care model involving a small number of providers, primarily nurses and contractual physicians; and 3) an off-site model. In the off-site model, routine initial health screening and management of minor ailments are provided at the facility by nonhealth care staff. Providers in the community usually perform physical examinations, evaluations, and emergency treatments off-site.

Despite the fact that the majority of incarcerated adolescents are enrolled in or eligible for state Medicaid-funded health care, this resource rarely is used to fund correctional health care programs. Federal Medicaid regulations still exclude incarcerated populations from Medicaid health care benefits. Some states and other local jurisdictions have chosen to interpret these regulations to allow Medicaid funding and Medicaid services to be provided to preadjudicated youths in short-term facilities. This has the potential to improve the level of care and offset the costs of health care programming.

Substandard Care

Despite decades of increased public attention, regulatory effort, scientific research, and litigation, significant improvements in juvenile correctional health care remain elusive. Surveys in the last five years have highlighted several problems:
- One-fifth of institutions do not provide sick call
- Two-fifths do not conduct medical screenings on admission
- One-fourth do not provide follow-up physical exams within the first week of confinement

- Half do not provide mental health care for youths
- Care for confined pregnant teenagers generally is inadequate

Health care standards for juvenile correctional facilities were initially established by the American Medical Association in 1979. The American Correctional Association and the National Commission on Correctional Health Care have health program accreditation procedures for juvenile correctional facilities, yet only a handful of state and local juvenile correctional facilities have been accredited.

Ethical Concerns

Traditionally, correctional health care has not always attracted medicine's best. Correctional health care professionals working in correctional settings routinely face difficult and complex situations, many of which arise from ethical questions, institutional policies, or funding constraints. A major concern in some institutions is that health care providers too often are asked to participate in practices that may adversely affect the health and well-being of youthful detainees. Such practices include the excessive use of disciplinary isolation and the misuse of mechanical or chemical restraints. Participation in practices that may have adverse health consequences raises legal and ethical dilemmas. (*See* "Making the Case for Bioethics in Corrections," page 55). In addition, medical personnel may be asked to perform body cavity searches to recover contraband or to obtain urine samples for drug screening.

Partnerships between juvenile correctional facilities and local health department providers or university medical school providers has improved care substantially in jurisdictions applying these models of care. An institution's ability to attract and retain well-trained health care professionals is a major element in providing adequate health care. In those partnerships with public health or academic medical training programs, health care trainees are sensitized to the health care needs of this population.

Summary

Experience tells us that health care organizations should become more involved in setting policies and providing health care within youth detention and correctional facilities. Public health departments in jurisdictions where these facilities exist should work to ensure that these facilities meet minimum standards of care. Facilities should adopt processes that ensure that systemwide goals and performance measures include health status measures for their inmate populations.

More and more health care professionals have become advocates for the health concerns of youths in correctional facilities, and several professional organizations have worked to improve services. These organizations include the Society for Adolescent Medicine, the American Bar Association, the Youth Law Center, the National Center for Youth Law, the American Medical Association, and the Maternal and Child Health Bureau of the Health Resources and Services Administration, as well as the American Correctional Association.

Juvenile correctional facilities, in collaboration with local health departments — or state institutions in collaboration with state public health programs and state Medicaid programs—should modify policies and regulations to permit full Medicaid coverage for youths who are otherwise eligible. For many local jurisdictions, the limiting step in providing comprehensive service is lack of financial resources.

Delinquent youths clearly represent an underserved population with many health care needs. Adolescents confined to correctional facilities should be protected as much as possible from developing physical and emotional problems that result from or are exacerbated by incarceration. Incarceration, even for short periods of time, should offer an opportunity for health screening and access. The hope is that these adolescents will become more productive and effective citizens through better health care and related rehabilitation programs.

References

Anderson, B. and J. A. Farrow. In press. Incarcerated Adolescents in Washington State: Health Services and Utilization. *Journal of Adolescent Health.*

Breuner, C. C. and J. A. Farrow. 1995. Pregnant Teens in Prison: Prevalence, Management and Consequences. *Western Journal of Medicine.*

National Commission on Correctional Health Care. 1995. *Standards for Health Services in Juvenile Detention and Confinement Facilities.* Chicago.

Meeting the Challenges of Juvenile Health Care

Thompson, L. S. Ed.. 1990. *The Forgotten Child in Health Care: Children in the Juvenile Justice System*. Washington, D.C.: National Center for Education in Maternal and Child Health.

Thompson, L. S. and J A. Farrow. 1993. Hard Time, Healing Hands. Arlington, Virginia: National Center for Education in Internal and Child Health.

∾

James Farrow, M.D., is director of adolescent medicine at the University of Washington in Seattle.

Addressing the Needs of Elderly Offenders

By Connie L. Neeley,
Laura Addison, and
Delores Craig-Moreland, Ph.D.

he U.S. Census Bureau reports that the elderly are the fastest-growing segment of the population—a statistic which already is reflected in the increase in elderly inmates in America's prisons. Inmates over the age of 50 will comprise 33 percent of the total prison population by the year 2010, says Judy Hudson, chief of nursing services for the Missouri Department of Corrections. "Inmates are serving more mandatory sentences and longer terms, and release policies are becoming more restrictive."

How can corrections accommodate this aging prison population? According to geriatric criminal specialists, most prisons are built for young offenders who are locked up, taught a trade, and sent back into society. But by the year 2000, an estimated 125,000 inmates will be 50 or older, and 35,000 of them will be over 65.

Corrections professionals must adopt proactive plans to provide for these elderly inmates, taking into consideration many elements of prison management, including balance and safety, humanitarian concerns, and money. Balance and safety issues include the basics of designing spaces that are accessible to the elderly. They should be equipped with smoke alarms, fire alarms, and sprinkler systems. The chief humanitarian concerns faced when managing elderly inmates involve keeping them in the workforce of the prison, giving them responsibility for parts of their lives, and helping them maintain family ties to strengthen their hold on reality. Medical and mental health issues address both humanitarian concerns and—because of the cost of caring for elderly inmates—financial considerations, as well.

Correctional facilities will have to stretch their budgets to accommodate this mushrooming number of aging inmates. A growing elderly prison population will be more costly to accommodate than a younger one because elderly inmates require more medical and mental health services in special settings.

Demographics

Older inmates are not a homogeneous group. Many variables influence their classification and management, including each one's health and personal background, criminal lifestyle, life experiences, relationships with family members and peers, and religious beliefs. Using a typology derived by geriatric criminal specialists Delores Craig-Moreland and William D. McLaurine Jr., elderly offender classifications can be broken down into four types: first-time offender, chronic offender, prison recidivist, and one who has grown old as an inmate.

A first-time offender in his fifties or sixties probably already is maladjusted in society and is poor at adapting to change. Sixty-one percent have committed sexual crimes. The first offender has a volatile personality that poses a risk for suicide, violence against other inmates, and has poor mental health. Such an inmate would benefit from living in a segregated setting with other older inmates.

A chronic offender has a propensity for criminal activity but has not been confined before. He is able to socialize with others and does not feel stigmatized by his criminal label. Serving a long sentence, with the prospect of dying in prison, causes a great deal of stress for this inmate, who is likely to be violent.

A prison recidivist usually adjusts well upon reentry because he already knows prison routine. He, too, has concerns about dying in prison and should be evaluated for potential health issues and supported in maintaining his self-respect. This inmate can be an asset in a separate living unit for older inmates. He can help first-time and chronic offenders adjust to prison life. An inmate who has grown old as an inmate also is an asset to the first two types, and is the least volatile in daily interactions. He has had meaningful activities and a work history while in prison.

Housing

Older inmates sometimes can present correctional facilities with housing conflicts. While correctional administrators try to house elderly inmates near
urban areas where medical specialists are available, these inmates often
express a desire to be closer to their families and so may resist a move to an
urban facility.

Older offenders do not like to be segregated or housed where their families
cannot visit, agrees McLaurine. Yet, these inmates do better when they are
away from the stress of interacting closely with younger offenders. Moving
them out of traditional areas and into specially constructed sections can free
up secure spaces needed for more violent inmates. Moving elderly inmates
also makes it easier for correctional officers to monitor their medical and
mental health needs.

Accessibility and safety are the two most important considerations in planning and designing housing for an aging prison population. Ramps and sub-
tle grades, with handrails where necessary, enhance access. Doors should be
three-feet wide, with thresholds one-half inch or lower. Levers should be used
in place of knobs, and the pulling force on door closers needs to be less than
five pounds.

Rick Holbrook, a justice facilities specialist, says existing spaces can be
remodeled to reflect changing needs. "You can retrofit existing facilities and
improve their conditions to meet ADA requirements, making them as barrier-
free as possible," he says. A geriatric unit consists of sleeping quarters that
can be made into a dormitory setting, with sleeping cubicles created by privacy screens. Holbrook recommends that each screened group not exceed
four inmates.

Restroom facilities can be provided at the ratio of one toilet and sink per
twelve male inmates, one per eight for females. Urinals can be substituted for
up to half of the toilets in the men's quarters. Showers also should be supplied
at a rate of one per eight inmates, and at least one bathtub should be provided. Grab bars are required in showers and tub areas, as well as for seats, and
flexible spray nozzles should be installed. The floor surfaces should be abra-
sive enough to minimize inmates slipping when the floor is wet.

Activities

Designing a comfortable environment to meet the needs of older inmates is an important part of helping them adjust to prison life. A day room in a prison geriatric unit should be a multipurpose space separate from the sleeping quarters. It can be a place for reading, playing games, watching television, talking, and dining.

Crafts and other activities should be encouraged to keep the older population active creatively, although a crafts room will need supervision. An examination room for routine checkups may double as a dispensary for medication, a counseling room, or an administrator's office. Keeping physical therapy in its own room will be a key component in helping older inmates stay healthy. Inmates also should have access to an outside recreational area for exercise, with shaded areas and drinking fountains that can be winterized.

Of course, all areas of the geriatric unit must be fully visible to staff members in the security post that is set up within it. "Typically, the older inmate is not a security problem and does not require a high-security cell," Holbrook says. "A dorm-type facility is adequate for older inmates." Such a minimum-security concept can bring costs down to approximately $100 per square foot, he adds, compared with $250 per square foot for a maximum-security prison.

Impaired eyesight requires good lighting, but not just brighter, bigger lights. A sensitivity to glare, which can affect balance, orientation, and memory span, also develops with age, so indirect lighting is more effective. Floor surfaces should not have high-gloss finishes or contrasting random patterns, and must be as nonslip as possible.

Sound control in day rooms can be accomplished with acoustical ceilings and low-pile carpets. The typical hard surfaces of detention facilities make it hard to distinguish one sound against a background of competing noises.

Medical Care

When older inmates take better care of themselves, they have fewer illnesses and make fewer trips to the infirmary. "It's essential to make the offender a partner in his or her health care through education on good health habits and compliance with treatment," says Missouri Department of Correction's Judy Hudson.

Keeping older inmates active is important. They should be offered activities that are practical for their ages and physical conditions, and should be allowed to keep reasonable assignments in the institutional workforce as a way of maintaining dignity and positive self-images. Older inmates who have some sense of control over their daily lives adjust better. In addition, helping them maintain their family ties will reinforce their links to reality as they age.

Bobbie Huskey, former president of the American Correctional Association, suggests that a different classification system be used to identify the medical needs of older inmates. Instead of declaring inmates elderly by chronological age, each category of this system should address a level of physical impairment with its different medical care needs, programs, and housing. Acute-care inmates have infectious diseases and require skilled nursing care. Extended care offers twenty-four-hour daily assisted living to those in the last stages of a terminal illness. Chronic care patients require daily access to health services, and to a medical unit if their mobility is severely restricted. Chronic, unstable patients also may require immediate access to health care for such services as dialysis. Chronic, stable patients are ambulatory and do not need to be in a special medical unit or separated from the general population.

According to Huskey, patients can move from category to category. For instance, after surgery or injury, an inmate may require daily nursing care or convalescent care in an infirmary, but only for a short period. After recovery, the inmate can be returned to a relatively self-sufficient life. Some inmates' frailty and restricted mobility require protective housing, but not round-the-clock nursing care. Prisons have increased their use of hospice care for terminally ill inmates in recent years, she adds.

Conclusion

In a time of increasingly longer prison sentences and decreasing resources for dealing with special prison populations, corrections professionals should practice proactive planning to address the rapidly growing elderly inmate population. Daily maintenance and attention are the best options in the long run. If the needs of the aging inmate population are neglected, it will create a more costly situation for the taxpayer down the road. According to Holbrook, everyone involved with housing prison populations needs to be involved in planning discussions with others in the field. "It's a proactive position on a major concern," he says. "We're all taxpayers."

~

Connie Neeley is a senior vice president for the architectural firm of Gossen Livingston Associates Inc. Laura Addison is a journalist in Wichita, Kansas. Delores E. Craig-Moreland, Ph.D., is assistant professor in the Department of Administration of Justice at Wichita State University.

Making a Case for Bioethics in Corrections

By Patricia N. Reams, M.D., M.P.H.,
Martha Neff Smith, Ph.D., John Fletcher,
and Edward Spencer, M.D.

J.W. is an HIV-positive inmate whose illness is progressing steadily. The infectious disease consultant recommends an expensive "cocktail" of medicines that are now J.W.'s only hope of survival. The warden warns that the prison cannot afford this treatment regimen. J.W. and his lawyer argue that he is entitled to health care in prison. Is J.W. entitled to these expensive medicines? What if paying for his treatment means that other prison programs must be cancelled? Is it in society's best interest to prolong J.W.'s life? Suppose J.W. is a convicted murderer serving a life sentence?

S.M. is an inmate who is suspected of concealing matches in her vagina. The warden asks the nurse to perform a pelvic examination. S.M. refuses to have the examination. Should the nurse force S.M. to undergo the examination? Does the nurse have a greater duty to her supervisor or to her patient? If she does not perform the examination, will her job be in jeopardy? If she does force it, will she be an effective health care provider for S.M. in the future? Can S.M. charge the nurse with assault? What if S.M. has threatened to harm herself or others with the matches?

The county jail recently has initiated a screening program for suicide. In reviewing the results, the psychologist realizes that many more inmates than previously had been suspected are at risk for suicide. He does not have the resources to counsel all of them adequately. Does he briefly interview all those at risk, knowing that his intervention will be insufficient? Does he select a few for more comprehensive treatment? How is the selection made?

Health care providers in correctional systems often face ethical dilemmas unlike those found in other medical settings (National Institute of Corrections, 1991). Issues of resource rationing, prisoners' rights, consent, confidentiality, and the providers' divided loyalties among patient, institution, and society create a unique environment for health care in corrections. Not only must those who deliver health care to inmates assure quality of care, but they also are charged with improving the efficiency of valuable health care resources while working in an institution which carries out society's goal of isolating, punishing, and rehabilitating offenders. When inmate litigation over alleged medical mistreatment is brought into the picture, the need for a bioethics program becomes clear.

A bioethics program is one which resolves issues related to the proper delivery of health care. Such a program provides policy recommendations based on ethical considerations; a practical means of resolving conflicts related to the ethics of providing health care; and a staff that is educated in the moral implications of health care decision making and objective measures of the effectiveness of the program. The program offers the potential for improved quality of care for inmates, creating greater satisfaction among inmates, staff, and administration. Care more often is delivered properly the first time, so expenses are reduced and potential lawsuits are avoided or more easily defended. A successful bioethics program ensures consensus among providers, administrators, and others regarding the proper delivery of health care, in compliance with established ethical principles and values.

The Ethics Movement

Minimum standards for health care in adult and juvenile correctional systems have been issued by the American Correctional Association and the National Commission on Correctional Health Care. They provide for autonomy in medical decision making and attempt to establish a philosophy that health care in prison systems should be equivalent to the community level of care. Although these standards have done much to improve the level of health care in correctional institutions, there are several problems with their content and application.

1. Because most correctional institutions are not certified by these national organizations, few are governed by the standards.

2. The standards emphasize procedural regularity without promoting performance, so compliance does not necessarily imply better care (Office of Juvenile Justice and Delinquency Prevention, 1994).

3. The standards are not as strict as current case law in some areas such as the participation of health care providers in isolation and restraint practices in juvenile institutions (Costello and Jameson, 1987).

4. The standards do not reflect a common perspective on ethical problems in prison systems.

5. The standards do not propose a method of deciding how ethical dilemmas should be resolved.

Correctional health care professionals must develop their own code of ethics to provide guidance on moral decision making or have them imposed by others, including courts, legislatures, employers, or third-party payers (Kipnis, 1990).

The American Correctional Health Services Association has developed a code of ethics for correctional health care providers. Its guiding principles are consistent with traditional professional standards of medical practice. Priorities of interest are ranked first for the individual patient, second for the health environment, and third for the security of the institution. Health providers are advocates for the needs of their patients. An ethics program would allow for the application of the American Correctional Health Services Association's code in individual institutions.

Ethical Considerations

Physicians, nurses, and other health care providers who work in prisons are bound by the same ethical considerations as their colleagues in the community. But, they face additional dilemmas because of their unique situation of practicing in a secure institution on patients whose rights are defined in a different context than patients in the community. Health care providers who work in prisons constantly must reevaluate their loyalty to their patients, the institution, and society as a whole. What follows is a discussion of some of the ethical questions common in correctional institutions.

Inmates' Rights — Upon imprisonment, an inmate forfeits several of his or her constitutional rights, including freedom of movement, the right to bear arms, freedom from search and seizure, and the ability to act on a life plan.

Although courts recognize that incarceration, by itself, does not deprive individuals of rights, the legitimate needs of the institution take precedence (Kay, 1991). Yet, the right to health care is guaranteed by the Eighth and Fourteenth Amendments to the Constitution. The Eighth Amendment provides, in part, that "cruel and unusual punishment (shall not be) inflicted." It is violated if correctional health care providers show "deliberate indifference" to a serious medical or psychiatric need. The Eighth Amendment most often is cited in cases of denied access to care or of interference with prescribed care. (Costello and Jameson, 1987 and Kay, 1991).

Case law, specifically *Youngberg v. Romeo*, has interpreted the Fourteenth Amendment "due process" clause as guaranteeing "minimally adequate" treatment, which often implies greater protection for inmates than that guaranteed under the Eighth Amendment (Costello and Jameson, 1987). Courts have interpreted the Eighth and Fourteenth Amendments as guaranteeing the rights of inmates to nutrition, shelter, and health care. Since most Americans do not have these rights, administrators and health care personnel may be ambivalent about the quantity and quality of care given.

Rationing—Rationing of care is a daily occurrence in a prison system. Prisons operate on tight budgets, and health care is expensive. Budget considerations may limit the number of health care providers and facilities, the number of patients who can be seen, or the adequacy of treatment. A provider, faced with limited resources, must decide if he or she gives adequate care to a few or inadequate care to many. A bioethics program could provide guidelines for appropriate health care distribution. Administrators and health care providers also may ration care to those whom they feel are least deserving of it. Some have questioned the sense in providing care to inmates on death row, for instance.

Others consider the length of a prisoner's sentence, the nature of the offense, and the perceived burden on society when deciding whether or not to pursue medical treatment. In addition, health care providers have been known to adopt the attitudes of inmates and delay or deny care for "manipulative behavior," such as attention-seeking behavior, or frequent or unfounded complaints (Rowan, 1989 and Start, 1988). A health care system must be designed to meet the needs of such patients. Therefore, health care providers who see such patients daily must have sufficient support, both intellectual and emotional, to perform their duties properly.

Confidentiality—Protection of patient privacy and confidentiality is problematic in a crowded prison. Although courts have upheld that an inmate has a right to privacy, it is not always possible. Some treatment programs, such as those for sex offenders or AIDS patients, carry a social stigma. If known to other inmates, the patient's safety could be in danger. A report by the National Institute of Corrections acknowledges the difficulty in protecting confidential information in a prison:

> In prisons, the public health imperatives and the need to protect others from illicit drugs or weapons may conflict more often with the health care practitioner's duty of confidentiality. Outside of prisons, providers do not practice in an alien surrounding; they do not have conflicting loyalties. Inside they do, and that ongoing tension affects how the principle of confidentiality is employed in practice (National Institute of Corrections, 1991).

Consent/Refusal—The principle of respect for autonomy is one of the basic principles of medical ethics. It is based on respect for persons and personal choices, and implies that a person may consent to treatment or refuse it. Freedom from restraint or coercion is necessary. If autonomy is dependent on the ability of a person to relate a moral decision to a chosen personal life plan, and placement in prison forfeits the ability to pursue a personal life plan, doubt clouds the application of the principle (Ackerman, 1991). Some scholars have argued that the nature of prisons precludes the ability of inmates to engage in informed consent. Others have stated that with adequate policies that support the inmate's ability to choose, "good enough" consent is possible (National Institute of Corrections, 1991). Informed consent requires that a patient be competent, that he or she understand the nature of the treatment to be given, and that he or she voluntarily decide to authorize the treatment. This implies a dialog between the provider and the patient based on trust. Trust is difficult if the inmate is aware of the provider's divided loyalties—to the patient and the institution.

"Free and informed consent" is not attainable when an inmate's privileges are dependent on participation in treatment. This is frequently the situation for inmates who have been incarcerated for sexual offenses or substance abuse (Greenland, 1988). The justice system may impose treatment as a condition of release. Inmates also have a right to refuse treatment. This becomes an issue when the health and safety of others is in jeopardy. Competent inmates have embarked on hunger strikes in order to achieve a goal, such as release from prison or better living conditions. Force-feeding under this condition could be considered an assault as was decided in the cases of *Schloendorff* v. *Society of New York Hospital and Natanson* v. *Kline* (Marshall, 1994).

On the other hand, Canadian courts have ruled that in some situations, treatment without consent is justified in order to preserve life. Since most hunger strike imbroglios are situation-specific, the outcome of ethical decision making may be different in each case (Kleinman, 1986). A bioethics program could guide the negotiation process in such situations.

Participation in Executions—Health care providers traditionally have been required to participate in carrying out the death penalty. The requirement to pronounce death may lead to complicity in the sentence if the inmate is still alive after a first attempt at execution and the means must be repeated. Since an inmate must be of sound mind to be executed, psychiatrists have been asked to prescribe medication to treat psychotic inmates so that the sentence may be completed. Health care providers may start intravenous lines, perform cut-downs, give technical advice, or prepare or administer lethal injections. The American Medical Association has declared that such participation by physicians is unethical (1993). The morality of physician participation in other aspects of the process of the death sentence, such as certifying the inmate's capacity to stand trial and determining sanity, also has been questioned (Miller, 1989 and Sargent, 1986).

On the other hand, some physicians have argued that if the death penalty is considered a terminal illness, it is the duty of the physician to provide humane care so that the inmate's sentence is carried out with as little pain as possible. (Hsieh, 1989). Others have noted that the death penalty is lawful because it is considered appropriate by a majority in a democratic society; it is society's "self-defense" (Martz, 1990). It can be argued that the physician has a duty to society to support its system of justice. Participation in the death penalty complies with the principle of "do no harm" if it deters crime or if it demonstrates compassion for the condemned. Thus, some physicians maintain that professional organizations should not rule on the morality of physician participation except to recommend that each physician exercise his or her own judgment after careful reflection. Physicians who are required to participate need guidance, such as would be provided by a bioethics program.

Participation in Institutional Practices—Health care providers may be called upon to participate in institutional practices that are harmful to the patient, such as the use of fixed restraints or the prescription of medications for behavior control. Inmates may be subjected to cavity searches, without consent, when they are suspected of harboring a weapon or an illegal substance. Although this is a security issue rather than a health care issue, health care providers may be called upon to perform the search. This may lead to problems with the patient-provider relationship if the provider is the same person who routinely cares for the inmate. However, it may be preferable to have the health care provider perform the search rather than an untrained correctional officer. A well-functioning bioethics program may provide guidelines for addressing when health care providers should be asked to perform searches.

Health Care System—Control over medical practice may be problematic in a correctional environment. The contract or position description outlines the health care provider's obligation to the institution; it seldom describes the obligation to the patient (Costello and Jameson, 1987). Providers may not be in control of screening practices for health care. For example, in some institutions, admitting staff do not screen for health needs, or they may not complete the neccessary forms. Untrained staff may administer medications or triage patients for health services. The NCCHC standards address this issue by stating that "matters of medical and dental judgment are the sole province of the responsible physician and dentist, respectively. However, security regulations applicable to facility personnel also apply to health personnel" (National Commission on Correctional Health Care, 1992).

Providers may not recognize, however, that institutional practices limit patients' access to them, or they may not understand their obligation to change their working conditions. This leaves them open to civil liability and to charges of violating the Eighth and Fourteenth Amendments (Costello and Jameson, 1987). A bioethics program would raise awareness of these issues and would provide a framework to resolve them.

Preventive Care — Inmates are at a greater risk of poor health than the general population. Poverty prior to incarceration, with lack of access to medical care, may have led to neglect of medical problems (Costello and Jameson, 1987). Crowded living conditions both before and during incarceration increase the risk of tuberculosis. (Centers for Disease Control, 1992). Incarceration presents an opportunity for preventive treatment that could enhance the future health of the inmates and forestall their likelihood of spreading diseases in the community after release.

A Bioethics Program

The issues discussed above are only a few of the problems that arise daily in prisons, jails, and in detention and juvenile centers. Others include terminal care in an uncaring environment, advance directives, the requirement to disclose HIV status, use of technology, and research on a vulnerable population. At the present time, there is no method of addressing these issues either in policy or on an individual basis. A process for determining the moral implications of these and other concerns should be available to all prison health care providers and administrators. What follows is a proposal for a bioethics program in a prison system that is based on the bioethics structure used in many hospitals (Center for Bioethics, University of Virginia).

Components of a bioethics program include a bioethics committee, a bioethics consultation service, education of staff, empirical investigations, and evaluation. These may be adapted to a prison system.

The Committee—The function of the traditional hospital ethics committee may be served by a health advisory committee that provides policy recommendations. It should be accountable to the administrative position or board that sets policy for the institution or the correctional system. The committee should serve as a forum for discussion of clinical ethical problems, and should make policy recommendations. The committee also should direct other aspects of the bioethics program, including the consultation service, education, networking, and evaluation. Advice given by the committee should be considered seriously but should not be binding on the institution or policymaking body. Institutional policy should assimilate the recommendations of the committee with the practical needs of the institution to forestall potential problems.

Its Makeup—So that the committee be able to operate objectively, without constraints by the exigencies of prison life, and so that recommendations reflect the values of the community, more than half the membership should consist of persons from outside the institution. Members should be selected from those with a background in ethics and be members of the clergy, lawyers, community health professionals, or other community leaders. Institutional representation on the committee should include health care and administrative staff. The chairperson of the committee is responsible for directing the activities of the group and for acting as a liaison between health care providers and prison administrators on ethical matters.

Education—The first item on the agenda of the committee should be its own education on ethical matters. Expert guidance may be needed at first. It would be helpful if a member of the committee had credentials in ethics. Otherwise, members may attend programs on hospital ethics or a consultant may be obtained. The services of a regional bioethics network may be helpful. Early topics should include an introduction to bioethics and ethical decision making, professional codes of ethics, autonomy and informed consent, confidentiality, rights of inmates, access to treatment, and the role of health professionals in a secure institution.

The second level of ethics education is for the health care and security staff. Case presentations and discussions at training sessions and institutional meetings may be a helpful and entertaining means of accomplishing this objective. To promote better relations with the community at large, invitations to the case presentations may be issued to community advisory groups or to those who live near the institution.

Consultation—Specific ethical questions may arise which require immediate attention and are beyond the scope of policy recommendations. Such situations require the services of an ethics consultant. The consultant should be one of a qualified, available team of well-trained individuals who have familiarity with the prison milieu. These individuals may be volunteers from the community or employees of the prison who have demonstrated a commitment to fair treatment of all concerned parties. The role of the consultant is to explicate the ethical facts, articulate the parameters of the case, and educate the persons involved in the situation. A recommendation for the resolution of each case should be made to the ethics committee following a clear discussion of the facts and specific issues.

Evaluation—Evaluation of the program is directed by the committee. Information and opinions should be sought from members of the health care staff, institutional administration, security staff, and the community. Evaluation should be conducted on a regular basis, with results shared throughout the institution.

Institutional Components

In addition to the bioethics program, other administrative components have been recommended to resolve many of the problems inherent in a system where security needs often conflict with the delivery of adequate health care. These components include a responsible physician who has the power to advocate for the health needs of inmates, appropriate nursing supervision by medical administrators, and a quality assurance program (Start, 1988).

Although there is overlap between the concept of a bioethics program and a quality assurance program, they are not the same. A bioethics program would promote good quality of care, but it would not oversee the quality assurance of the health care system. A bioethics program would include persons from outside the prison system and provide nonbinding discussion and recommendations for the proper delivery of health care. The quality assurance program would be composed of persons who deliver care within the prison system and are in a position to change any noted deficiencies.

The bioethics program need not incur a great monetary cost to the institution. Community representatives on the committee may serve voluntarily, or with no more reimbursement than travel costs. Membership in a regional bioethics network may provide access to educational and consultation services.

A benefit of the program should be a better understanding of the relationship between security and health care staff. Whereas the prevailing ethos of the physician-patient relationship is one of mutual trust and respect, that of a correctional institution is hierarchical and controlling. Health care providers must be constantly vigilant to prevent a shift in their own attitudes toward that of the institution (National Institute of Corrections, 1991). At the same time, administrators and staff should understand that the role of health care providers includes advocacy for the health care needs of their patients.

A bioethics program, as structured above, potentially has great value for a correctional institution or system. It would promote quality medical care, support health care staff in ethical decisions, and elevate the level of understanding between health care and administrative staff. Policies based on ethical principles can only benefit the institution and those incarcerated behind its walls.

References

Ackerman, T. F. 1991. "Why Doctors Should Intervene." *In Biomedical Ethics, 3rd Edition*. T. A. Mappes and J. S. Zembaty, editors. New York: McGraw-Hill, Inc.

American Medical Association Council on Ethical and Judicial Affairs. 1993. "Physician Participation in Capital Punishment.." *Journal of American Medical Association*. 270: (3): 365- 368.

Centers for Disease Control. 1992. *Control of Tuberculosis in Correctional Facilities*. Washington, D.C.: Government Printing Office.

Costello, J. D. and J. J. Jameson. 1987. "Legal and Ethical Duties of Health Care Professionals to Incarcerated Children." *Journal of Legal Medicine*. 8:191-263.

Faiver, K. 1998. *Health Care Management Issues in Corrections*. Lanham, Maryland: American Correctional Association.

Greenland, C. 1988. "The Treatment and Maltreatment of Sexual Offenders: Ethical Issues." *Annual of New York Academy of Science*. 528:373-378.

Hsieh, D. S. 1989. "Physicians Should Give Injections." *Journal of the American Medical Association*. 261(1): 132.

Kay, S. L. 1991. "The Constitutional Dimensions of an Inmate's Right to Health Care." Chicago: National Commission on Correctional Health Care.

Kipnis, K. 1990. "Professional Ethics in correctional Health Services: Clearing the Ground." *Corhealth*. October/November.

Kleinman, I. 1986. "Force Feeding: The Physician's Dilemma." *Canadian Journal of Psychiatry*. 31: 313-316.

Marshall, M. F.1994. "When the Patient Refuses Treatment." In *Introduction to Clinical Ethics*. J. C. Fletcher, C. B. Hite and P. A. Lombardo, editors. Charlottesville, Viriginia: University of Virginia.

Martz, E. W. 1990. "Society's Self-Defense." *Delaware Medical Journal*. 62(11): 138.

Making a Case for Bioethics in Corrections

Miller, A. M. 1989. "Amnesty International Stands Opposed." *Journal of the American Medical Association*. 261(1): 132-133.

National Commission on Correctional Health Care. 1992. *Standards for Health Services in Juvenile Detnetion and Confinement Facilities*. Chicago: National Commission on Correctional Health Care.

National Institute of Corrections. 1991. *Prison Health Care: Guidelines for the Management of an Adequate Delivery System*. Chicago: National Commission on Correctional Health Care.

Office of Juvenile Justice and Delinquency Prevention. 1994. Conditions of Confinement: Juvenile Detention and Corrections Facilities. Cambridge, Massachusetts: Abt Associates, Inc.

Rowan, J. 1989. "Street Attitudes of Health Care Providers Promote Lawsuits." *Corhealth*. March/April/May.

Sargent, D. A., 1986. "Treating the Condemned to Death." *Hastings Center Report*. December. 16(6): 5-6.

Start, A. H. 1988. "Correctional Health Care Programs Properly Administered." *Corrections Today*. February.

≈

Patricia N. Reams, M.D., M.P.H., is a pediatrician at Cumberland Hospital for Children and Adolescents in New Kent, Virginia, and former chief physician for the Department of Juvenile Justice in Virginia. Martha Neff Smith, Ph.D., is on the faculty in public health and nursing at the Johns Hopkins University. John Fletcher, Ph.D., is director of the Center for Biomedical Ethics at the University of Virginia. Edward Spencer, M.D., is director of outreach programs at the Center for Biomedical Ethics.

Integrating Substance Abuse and Domestic Violence Treatment

By Stephen V. Valle, Sc.D., Nick Demos, J.D., Raymond Broaddus, Ph.D., William Mango, Lorraine Cohen, Monroe Parrot, and Bruce Fry, J.D.

he relationship between substance abuse and crime is well documented. Our nation's prisons and jails are filled with offenders in need of substance-abuse treatment. According to the Bureau of Justice Statistics (1992), more than two-thirds of violent offenders report that either they or their victims were using alcohol or drugs at the time of the crime. In New York state alone, more than 80 percent of the prison population has been identified as having substance-abuse problems.

On the other hand, almost a quarter of the inmates serving time for homicide or assault, and a third of those sentenced for sexual assault, were convicted of attacking a relative or an intimate such as an ex-spouse, boyfriend, or girlfriend. Another one-third reported that they knew their victims. According to the American Psychological Association (1996), approximately four million American women are beaten annually by current and former male partners. Domestic violence against women causes more injuries than automobile accidents, muggings, and rapes combined (Bureau of Justice Statistics, 1992).

Statistics on the prevalence of domestic violence are staggering. Nearly one-fourth of women in the United States will be abused by a current or former domestic partner within their lifetimes (American Medical Association, 1992). Battered women comprise 20 to 30 percent of women seeking care in emergency rooms (Hyman, et al. 1995); 14 to 28 percent of female ambulatory care patients; 23 percent of women seeking prenatal care; 25 percent of women presenting for psychiatric emergency care; and 64 percent of female patients admitted for inpatient psychiatric services (Warshaw, 1993).

Moreover, studies have shown that the average woman is assaulted thirty-five times before contacting the police (Bain, 1989).

While domestic violence often is associated with substance-related disorders, not all batterers are substance abusers (Resnick, 1994). And studies have shown that while substance abuse and violent behavior frequently coexist, the violent behavior will not end unless interventions address the violence as well as the addiction.

The New York State Substance Abuse/Domestic Violence prison therapeutic community is the first program to address both substance abuse and domestic violence in a prison setting. While the program has documented some initial success, its long-term viability will depend largely on the ability of correctional administrators to face the challenges inherent in implementation.

The CASAT Program

The rationale for establishing substance-abuse treatment services within the New York Department of Correctional Services had its origins in the early 1980s. At that time, administrators recognized that an intervention program for incarcerated offenders would have a strong impact on reducing recidivism, resulting in an overall cost reduction for the taxpayer.

According to the New York Department of Correctional Services, during the last twenty-five years, the number of drug offenders committed to state prisons in New York has grown dramatically—from 470 in 1970 to more than 10,000 annually from 1991 through 1995. In 1996, the number of drug commitments dipped slightly to 9,841. Approximately 74 percent of offenders under custody in New York report using drugs prior to incarceration or are classified as alcoholics based on the Michigan Alcohol Screening Test. Nationwide, 43 percent of state prison inmates report using drugs daily in the months prior to the offense for which they are incarcerated (New York Department of Correctional Services, 1996).

The New York 1989 Prison Omnibus Legislation provided for the expansion of existing alcohol and substance-abuse treatment programs administered by the New York Department of Correctional Services. The legislation called for the establishment of six 200-bed alcohol and substance-abuse treatment annexes at specific locations. Persons successfully completing the annex phase of treatment would be transferred to a work-release facility or an appropriate community-based program. The law also provided for an after-care component to be provided upon release from the department while under supervision of the Division of Parole. These legislative requirements resulted in the creation of the Comprehensive Alcohol and Substance Abuse Treatment program (CASAT). The CASAT program is intended to provide a continuum of treatment services designed to achieve the following goals:

- To better prepare participants for return to their families and communities
- To focus facility resources on the needs of inmates with a history of alcohol and substance abuse
- To ensure appropriate aftercare services in the community
- To increase coordination among pertinent state and local agencies, service providers, and community organizations
- To reduce drug and alcohol relapse and recidivism rates for program participants

The CASAT program consists of three phases. The first phase involves participation in an Alcohol and Substance Abuse Correctional Treatment Center (ASACTC)—a medium-security facility, which operates as a therapeutic community. Treatment focuses on chemical dependency and includes drug education, counseling programs, and the development of skills and coping mechanisms to facilitate recovery. The activities in the annex are designed to prepare residents to participate in phase II, the community reintegration phase, and phase III, aftercare. New York's implementation of in-prison substance-abuse treatment services supplemented by contractual agreements with community-based providers has enhanced greatly its ability to address inmates' addiction problems and has freed up prison beds for violent offenders.

Program Development

The New York Department of Correctional Services has a long and highly regarded history of providing innovative substance-abuse treatment programs for offenders. New York also was the first state in the nation to establish a permanent, statutory agency dedicated exclusively to domestic violence. The New York State Office for the Prevention of Domestic Violence was established in 1992, and is responsible for strengthening the state's responses to domestic violence.

In 1993, the Center for Substance Abuse Treatment announced the availability of $12.5 million to support demonstration projects under the "Model

Comprehensive Substance Abuse Treatment Programs for Correctional Populations" initiative. Under this initiative, New York received a three-year, $1.95 million grant to establish an intensive therapeutic community treatment program for domestic-violence offenders with substance-abuse problems. When the grant money expired in 1996, New York continued to fund the program at its grant level of $650,000 per year.

In awarding the grants, the Center for Substance Abuse Treatment recognized that the demonstration projects would need a wide range of technical assistance. Even demonstration projects situated in correctional systems with a strong history of providing drug treatment services can experience operational start-up difficulties, community and organizational resistance to new program approaches, and other barriers in implementing programs. That same year, the Center for Substance Abuse Treatment contracted with Johnson, Bassin & Shaw Inc. to provide technical assistance and training services to the demonstration prison drug-treatment programs in prison.

During its three-year developmental period, the New York program experienced significant challenges from both the internal and external environments, including frequent turnover among direct-care staff and changes in the administration of the correctional facility. To assist the program during this period, the Center for Substance Abuse Treatment provided ongoing technical assistance which focused on reviewing and assessing the program's progress in meeting its stated goals and objectives. The mentoring role provided by the technical assistance consultant proved to be an invaluable asset to the program as it progressed through the developmental stages, and is considered one of the key ingredients in the success of the program.

The New York Program

The Substance Abuse/Domestic Violence program at New York's Eastern Correctional Facility Annex, a medium-security facility located in Ulster County, New York, is a six-month program for up to 180 male offenders with histories of domestic-violence and substance-abuse problems. The goal of the project is to develop integrated substance-abuse and domestic-violence treatment services in the context of a therapeutic-community structure.

The staffing pattern consists of three treatment teams of alcohol and substance-abuse counselors, one team for each of the sixty-bed dorms. A senior counselor supervises the treatment staff. All staff also received training in both substance-abuse treatment and domestic violence prior to the commencement of the program. Ongoing cross-training and specialized team-building and therapeutic-community skills training have occurred throughout the duration of the program. In an effort to create an integrated curriculum, all counselors receive continuous training in domestic-violence intervention, as well as the 12-step model of substance-abuse treatment.

The treatment program includes peer training and supervision, community meetings, Alcoholics Anonymous and Narcotics Anonymous meetings, group counseling, individual counseling, lectures, and specialized treatment groups. Participants are enrolled in three hours of treatment, three hours of education, and three hours of work per day, five days a week. If education is not needed, residents may work an additional three hours per day. In addition, residents participate in self-help programs and personal assignments during nonprogram hours.

The philosophy of the program is that addiction and domestic violence are viewed as "power and control" defenses which must be addressed simultaneously, as the exhibition of either behavior is likely to trigger addiction relapse and/or renewed acts of domestic violence. Continued abstinence from all mood-altering chemicals, as well as ongoing modification of violent behavior, are necessary for continued successful recovery.

During the fourth month of the six-month program, residents complete an aftercare plan which includes enrollment in a community-treatment program, employment and/or vocational training, making living arrangements, developing a schedule of daily self-help meetings, and attending weekly domestic-violence classes.

Varied Philosophies

In addition to dealing with the normal challenges of starting a new treatment program within the structure of a prison setting, several other obstacles to implementation were identified, the first of which was the need to integrate therapeutic community, domestic violence, and substance abuse philosophical perspectives into one cohesive program.

While the therapeutic community model has been around since the 1960s, it is only recently that the therapeutic community concept has been accepted widely in correctional settings as the preferred mode of treatment for offenders with substance-abuse problems. This is due, in part, to the overwhelmingly positive research that has demonstrated that offenders who complete a therapeutic community program have better outcome results than offenders who receive no treatment, or those who participate in other treatment modalities.

The traditional therapeutic community model of the 1960s and 1970s had been criticized in some professional circles as being overly dependent upon a charismatic leader; prone to being cultist in nature; and ambivalent regarding abstinence from alcohol for drug addicts. It also was criticized for practicing behavior change tactics that were viewed as degrading, punitive, and humiliating. In contrast, the modified therapeutic community model currently incorporated in many prison programs has integrated aspects of traditional addiction treatment and recent advances in offender-outcome studies.

A modified prison-based therapeutic community model generally includes the following standards:
- Use of cognitive-behavioral strategies for behavior change and life-skills acquisition
- Insistence upon abstinence from all drugs, including alcohol, as a prerequisite for program participation, and a strong emphasis on accountability
- Incorporation of self-help models in the program structure
- Greater emphasis on positive reinforcement and affirmation of the individual. Learning experiences that are humiliating and disrespectful are not acceptable in today's more effective therapeutic community model

The introduction of domestic-violence offenders into a substance-abuse therapeutic-community model added an additional philosophical variable that needed to be integrated. This was a major challenge for the program, as there were no previous prison-based models that simultaneously treated domestic violence and substance abuse.

The domestic-violence intervention model used most often in community settings is principally a pro-feminist model. It is essential, in this model, to challenge the sexist expectations and controlling behaviors that underlie violent behavior toward women. Power and control are seen as the fundamental issues to be addressed. Interventions challenge the abusive man's attempts to control his partner through the use of physical force, verbal and nonverbal intimidation, and psychological abuse. Rather than viewing battering as a skill deficit or a stress-management problem, this model views battering as a sexist control problem.

Core principles found in traditional addiction treatment, including powerlessness, loss of control, and denial, are challenged and viewed as rationalizations to avoid responsibility for one's sexist control problem. Compounding the philosophical differences was the culture clash that exists between the male-dominated, authoritarian, and perceived punitive nature of a correctional environment, and that of a pro-feminist philosophy and culture of domestic-violence counselors.

Treatment

The challenges of integrating a substance-abuse treatment culture into a correctional environment are significant. As treatment programs and training initiatives in correctional settings have become more common, substance-abuse professionals have learned that treatment cannot be effective in an environment where treatment and security are at cross purposes. As a result of this experience, treatment professionals have learned to respect the invaluable role that security plays in creating a safe environment for treatment; understand and work within the structure of an authoritarian organization; and be vigilant about maintaining clear boundaries in relationships with inmates.

Substance-abuse professionals have learned over time how to work within the limitations provided in a correctional setting, and to view the structure of a correctional system as an added therapeutic tool. For example, whereas coercion at one time was viewed by treatment professionals as being antitherapeutic, it now is regarded generally as a legitimate therapeutic tool to motivate resistant clients. Thus, substance-abuse treatment professionals, through extensive training and cross-training efforts, not only have learned to coexist with security staff, but have learned to view corrections professionals as allies and partners in treatment.

Providers of domestic-violence treatment, however, have not had years of experience working in a prison setting. Most domestic-violence programs are in the community and take place in an environment under the control of the providers. It became apparent that the cultural clashes between a pro-feminist domestic-violence model, a male-dominated corrections culture, and a prison-based modified therapeutic community substance-abuse treatment culture were significant. Because the pro-feminist domestic-violence provider was not able to grasp the necessity of accommodating the corrections and substance-abuse cultures, the domestic-violence vendor ultimately was removed as an on-site provider. However, much of the core content of the model was retained; training and consulting were made available; and the content of the domestic-violence program gradually was integrated into the substance-abuse program.

From this experience, it became apparent that there are many complementary and integrative elements among the domestic violence, substance abuse, corrections, and therapeutic community paradigms. This has led to the evolution of an integrative approach that addresses domestic violence within the context of an abstinence-based and crime-free lifestyle. Some of the integrative elements we learned from this program include the following:

- Team-building and continual cross-training are essential ingredients in forging an integrative approach to substance abuse and domestic violence. Team-building that stresses the exploration of attitudes in an experiential rather than solely content-based format is important.
- A corrections approach to program services should be multidimensional and involve other disciplines, such as education, medicine, work assignments, and so forth. Treatment professionals often minimize the importance of these requirements, which creates divisions among security and treatment staff.
- Security and treatment staff should search for common ground, even while following what appear at first to be incompatible philosophies.
- Staff should receive clinical supervision to help them integrate new ideas and conceptual models for changing behavior. Clinical supervision should be provided by an individual who is not involved in the day-to-day operations of the program. The content of clinical supervision should be confidential to allow for staff to explore changing attitudes in safety.

Staff Challenges

This new integrated program model requires a staff with a broad background in the various program elements. Unfortunately, few professional counselors have such a background. For an established program with a core group of experienced staff, this may not be as great an obstacle, but for a new model, it was a significant limiting factor. The program was able to adjust to this limitation by enhancing training opportunities for staff and by using technical assistance provided by the Center for Substance Abuse Treatment.

The development of a therapeutic community program in a correctional setting follows a normal developmental process that often is characterized by considerable turmoil, staff changes, and uncertainty, until such time as the therapeutic community culture is fully integrated into the prison setting. It is not uncommon for this developmental process to take up to two or three years before a program reaches a maturation stage where the therapeutic community is operating in a stable and routine manner. The three developmental stages for a prison therapeutic-community program that we identified are as follows:

Stage One: This stage usually lasts for most of the first year, and is characterized by frequent changes in the staff, power, and control struggles among correctional and treatment staff, role confusion for both the correctional and treatment staff, instability in the peer hierarchy, and frequent changes in the design and operation of the therapeutic-community program. It is important for program administrators and managers to exhibit patience during the first year, not to have unrealistic expectations during this stage, and not to be alarmed at temporary periods of chaos and instability.

Stage Two: This stage is characterized by a period of testing and challenging of the therapeutic-community structure by the professional staff (custody and civilian), as well as the inmate population. Continual cross-training and clinical supervision are critical variables during this stage. The program starts to stabilize as new material is integrated into the original core design and peer leadership starts to flourish. Program detractors either are phased out or their influence is minimized. Opposition from resistant security staff usually is neutralized as strong support from the majority of the security staff emerges.

Stage Three: This stage is characterized by a gradual acceptance of the therapeutic-community structure and peer-hierarchy concept by the inmate population as well as the staff, increasingly prolonged periods of program stabilization, and an eventual period of program maturation. Staff turnover and challenges to the therapeutic-community concept are considerably reduced as the therapeutic-community culture replaces the inmate culture.

Effective Programming

Several principles were identified as essential ingredients for programs treating offenders with histories of substance abuse and domestic violence.

- Cross-Training of Treatment and Security Staff: It is essential that initial cross-training of security and treatment staff be conducted before inmates enter the program, and at regular intervals during the first few years of a program. This training needs to focus on attitudes, values, and perceptions relating to addictions, public safety, corrections, public health, and personal experience with people who have alcohol and drug problems. The content of cross-training is important, but less important than exploration of attitudes and activities that focus on team-building. Such cross-training events should take place at least once a year after a program is mature, and more frequently during earlier developmental stages.
- Technical Assistance Consultation and Training: The importance of having technical assistance available to programs that address substance abuse and domestic violence is critical for a program's ability to address barriers and conflicts that inevitably will emerge. The technical assistance consultant should be from outside the agency and possess a wide range of technical, interpersonal, and professional skills.
- Program Evaluation: Both process and outcome evaluation components are important program design elements. The evaluators should be integrated into the team to enhance the effectiveness of the evaluation process. It is important to recognize that the initial evaluation process should focus on process evaluation variables. Actual data collection for outcome purposes should begin only after the first year of operations.
- Flexibility in Selecting Personnel: The key to an effective treatment program is the quality of personnel who deliver direct-care services. Administrators need to be able to have the flexibility to select staff who not only possess the necessary professional skills, but who also have personal qualities that foster team-building and adaptability. The ability to hire and terminate personnel without hindrance is an important variable in developing a cohesive staff.
- Support of Host Facility Administrators: In establishing prison-based treatment programs, it is vital that support of the facility administration and security staff be obtained. This can be facilitated by involving facility superintendents/wardens in the planning process before programs are implemented, and by keeping them informed.

Conclusion

The New York State Department of Corrections Substance Abuse/Domestic Violence Treatment Program has proven that domestic violence and substance abuse can be treated successfully in a prison-based modified therapeutic community structure. However, managers and decision makers must be aware of the many challenges that will arise when implementing such a dual-disorder program, and have strategic plans for addressing these challenges. By following the principles that were developed in the New York model and by learning from this experience, programs are more likely to be successful.

References

American Medical Association, Council on Ethical and Judicial Affairs. 1992. Physicians and Domestic Violence: Ethical Considerations. *Journal of the American Medical Association*. 267 (23):3190-3193.

———. 1992. Diagnostic and Treatment Guidelines on Domestic Violence. Chicago: Reprinted in *Archives of Family Medicine* 1(1):39-47.

American Psychological Association. 1996. Violence and the Family. Report of the Association Presidential Task Force on Violence and the Family. Washington, D.C.

Bain, J. 1989. Spousal Assault: The Criminal Justice System and the Role of the Physician. *Ontario Medical Review*. (December) 56(1):20-28,49.

Bureau of Justice Statistics. Drugs, Crime and the Justice System. 1992 Washington, D.C.: Bureau of Justice Statistics. (December).

Hyman, et. al. 1995. Laws Mandating Reporting of Domestic Violence: Do They Promote Patient Well-Being? *Journal of the American Medical Association*. 273:22, 1781. June.

Irons, R. 1996. Co-morbidity Between Domestic Violence and Addictive Disease. In *Sexual Addiction and Compulsivity* 3(2):88-96.

New York Department of Correctional Services. 1996. *The Comprehensive Alcohol and Substance Abuse Treatment Program Manual*. June. Albany, New York.

Resnick, P. J. 1994. Profiles in Violence: Predictors of Violence. *Audio-Digest Family Practice*. 42(32)(side A & B):August.

Warshaw, C. 1993. Domestic Violence. Challenges to Medical Practice. *Journal of Women's Health* 2(1):73-79.

Wexlar, H., J. Blackmore, and D. Lipton. 1991. Project Reform: Developing a Drug Abuse Treatment Strategy for Corrections. *Journal of Drug Issues.* Spring. 21(2):469-490.

↡

Stephen K. Valle, Sc.D., is president of American Criminal Justice Solutions Inc., and Adcare Recovery Services Inc. in Boston; Nick Demos, J.D., is chief of the Systems Development and Integration Branch for the Substance Abuse and Mental Health Services Administration (SAMHSA); Raymond Broaddus, Ph.D., is deputy commissioner of the New York Department of Correctional Services; William Mango is assistant deputy commissioner of the New York Department of Correctional Services; Lorraine Cohen is senior correctional counselor for the New York Department of Correctional Services; Monroe Parrott is a correctional counselor for the New York Department of Correctional Services; and Bruce Fry, J.D., is a principal with Johnson, Bassin & Shaw in Silver Spring, Maryland.

Therapeutic Communities:

History, Effectiveness, and Prospects

By Douglas S. Lipton, Ph.D.

even out of every ten men and eight out of every ten women in the criminal justice system are drug users—persons who used illicit drugs with some regularity prior to entering the criminal justice system (Belenko and Peugh, 1998; Prendergast, Wellisch, and Falkin, 1995). The Federal Drug Use Forecasting system data show that the use of all drugs except cocaine has increased since 1989, and cocaine remains at the same level (Lipton, 1997). Accordingly, the 1990s have seen major increases in arrests of drug users, followed by pressure for funds to expand correctional capacity to treat those inmates with serious drug problems. Interestingly, with this increase has come increased public support for programs aimed at treating drug users and curbing drug-related crime. There is a genuine public and government concern that without treatment, most drug-involved offenders will resume their criminal activities and drug use after release and inevitably will return to criminal justice system custody.

The 1994 Crime Bill included, for the first time, a substantial sum provided for treatment of inmates in state and local correctional systems. The Residential Substance Abuse Treatment for State Prisoners Formula Grant Program (abbreviated RSAT) legislation created an opportunity for states to apply for funds to establish residential substance-abuse programs beginning in 1996. In conjunction with this legislation, Congress has authorized spending $270 million for the first five years of the program, the largest sum ever for the development and enhancement of substance-abuse treatment programs in state and local correctional facilities.

Largely because of research showing that prison-based therapeutic community programs significantly can reduce recidivism and drug relapse, RSAT legislation encourages the development of this residential treatment model, in addition to other viable treatment approaches, including cognitive-skills training, behavioral programming, vocational methods, and even 12-step programming.

Therapeutic Communities

Historically, the term "therapeutic community" has been used for several different forms of treatment—sanctuaries, residential group homes, and even special schools—and for several different conditions, including mental illness, drug abuse, and alcoholism. For example, the British therapeutic community emerged primarily as a process for treating military veterans as they returned from WW II with serious neurotic conditions from their experiences in combat and as prisoners of war. The term was coined when Thomas Main pioneered a therapeutic model combining community therapy with ongoing psychoanalytic psychotherapy in 1946. This was a modification of therapeutic work developed about the same time by Maxwell Jones and several others. By 1954, therapeutic community ideas were influencing wards in British psychiatric hospitals.

At about the same time, the use of tranquilizers began to emerge as the dominant "treatment" for institutionalized, mentally disordered persons. Drastic reductions in psychiatric beds and other confinement beds occurred as facilities closed down. In the 1950s and 1960s, the therapeutic-community movement shifted toward other milieus, notably corrections, and therapeutic community principles began to guide offender programs in the United Kingdom. Grendon Prison was built in 1959 specifically with a number of wings within which therapeutic communities would operate experimentally to provide treatment for psychologically disturbed offenders.

The British prison therapeutic communities operate within these principles:
- enfranchisement and empowerment, "wherein every community member has a direct say in every aspect of how the wing is run" (including the power to vote someone out for breach of a rule)
- a philosophy of tolerance to allow members to make mistakes, and to accept themselves "with all their warts" and support each other "regardless of their warts"

- encouragement of individual and especially collective responsibility and accountability
- continuous, direct, and candid presentation of interpretations of one another's behavior to counteract any tendency to distort, deny, or withdraw from interpersonal difficulties or rule breaking
- peer group influence, used to control and modify inimical prison cultural values with an important role for "community elders"—members who have successfully completed the transition themselves and who now play a supportive role.

Therapeutic goals include: getting past denial; relieving of intrapsychic distress; developing relationships with women and children, authority figures, and one another; changing attitudes toward offending, and specifically to one's primary offense; building morality, victim awareness, contrition, and understanding of effects on victims; and using relapse prevention techniques. At HMP Grendon, the treatment program lasts for more than two years, and consists of daily small therapy groups of ten residents run by two staff members (one psychologist and one trained officer); daily community "wing" meetings of thirty-five to forty-two (and as many as fifty); "feedbacks" or confrontation sessions; and cognitive skills, psychodrama, social and life skills, alternatives to violence, and educational programming.

In the United States

American therapeutic-communities have a different origin. They tend to be for drug-dependent and drug-abusing persons and derive from Synanon, which was both a social movement and a program founded in 1958 by Charles Dederich, a recovered alcoholic who, unfulfilled by Alcoholics Anonymous, founded his own racially integrated community of former addicts and ex-offenders. Synanon consisted, in part, of a kind of group therapy with intense emotional catharsis-type participation sessions; fairly "brutal" confrontation sessions; educational seminars; and discussions, not of drugs, but of self-image, work habits, and self-reliance. Synanon, which got its name when a newly arrived addict confused the terms "seminar" and "symposium," bears many similarities to today's Phoenix House and Daytop Village programs, although these programs tend to be considerably less intense.

Therapeutic Communities

The United States therapeutic-community model is less psychoanalytical and psychotherapeutic than the United Kingdom model. It is less focused on the criminal offense or on substance abuse per se and is more holistic, that is, more concerned with lifestyle changes across more dimensions. The United States model uses the "community of peers" and role models as change agents rather than professional clinicians and trained correctional officers, and it is less democratic in operation and more hierarchical in structure. The United States model also is less psychiatric (and less medical) in origin, emerging from a recovered client self-help background. Thus, American therapeutic communities (also called concept-based therapeutic communities) generally subscribe to a self-help, social-learning model approach and a holistic-human change perspective.

In 1969, the first correctional therapeutic community that served as a model program began in the federal penitentiary in Marion, Illinois. The prison psychiatrist, Dr. Martin Groder, designed and developed a therapeutic community based on his transactional analysis training and group therapy experience in California. The program combining these two general approaches was named "Aesklepieian" for the Greek god of healing, and consisted of intensive group counseling using the "community" or peer group as the vehicle for change, combined with the concepts and language of transactional analysis. While it did not meet the criteria we now have for this kind of treatment, it still served as a model for the development of correctional-based therapeutic communities in federal and several state institutions in the early and mid-1970s.

With the availability of Federal Law Enforcement Assistance Administration funds in the 1970s, even more prison therapeutic community programs were developed. For example, between 1975 and 1977, four institutions in Arkansas developed prison-based therapeutic communities, including one for female offenders; all were discontinued in 1980. Eight therapeutic communities began in Connecticut about the same time for persons addicted to drugs. Connecticut also established a therapeutic community for women at Niantic and one for juveniles at Cheshire, as well as several community-based correctional therapeutic communities. None of these programs followed the Aesklepieian model, but adapted the Daytop treatment model, which was much closer to the current prison-based therapeutic community model than Aesklepieian.

A therapeutic community was established in the Atlanta Penitentiary in Georgia in 1982, but was closed down in 1985 because of staff burnout and a lack of fresh volunteers. A therapeutic community for women was established in Michigan in 1977, moved to a smaller facility in 1982 and closed down in 1984, but reopened in 1988 and continues today. Missouri launched a therapeutic community for sex offenders in 1981. Close examination reveals that while separated from other inmates, members never established a community structure and were dispersed to the general population in 1988.

For five years, from 1979 to 1984, Nebraska ran a therapeutic community at Lincoln, but it closed after encountering a variety of problems, including friction between program staff and institutional staff, a negative investigative article by a reporter, crowding, and declining state revenues. In 1979, Florida developed the Lantana therapeutic community for youthful offenders, which was cited as an exemplary program by the federal government. It lasted until 1987, by which time it had lost energy and focus.

Successful Programs

Using the community-based drug abuse treatment program of Phoenix House as a model, the Stay'n Out program began in 1977 in New York. It is still operating quite successfully as a treatment program, and now has 5 units treating 180 men at Arthur Kill Correctional Facility, and about 40 women at Bayview Correctional Facility. The staffing is contracted out and still consists mainly of recovered, formerly addicted, ex-offenders. The cost per year, per inmate participant is less than $3,000. Stay'n Out has lasted longer than most correctional programs, in part, because it has developed strong ties to the political and academic communities; educated and cultivated both substance abuse and correctional administration officials, as well as line officers; encouraged careful and thoughtful long-term evaluation; and informed the public of its activities and accomplishments through the media.

Oklahoma began six small therapeutic communities in 1973, one of which was for drug offenders. All six were closed in 1979 when their primary proponent retired. The institution in which they were housed was torn down, and replaced with a new reception center. Oregon's Cornerstone program, a thirty-two bed therapeutic community for inmates that began in 1975, closed in 1996. A concept-based therapeutic community like Stay'n Out, Cornerstone differed by employing a higher proportion of professional staff and trained correctional officers than Stay'n Out. Thus, the cost of treatment at Cornerstone was greater than at Stay'n Out. Cornerstone's cost per day, per participant at the time of its closing had reached $39, making its cost comparable to that of some community-based therapeutic communities.

A therapeutic community was started in 1975 in South Carolina; it lasted until 1979, by which time it had become crowded, corrupted with contraband drugs, and inadequately staffed. In Virginia, a therapeutic community called House of Thought was established on the Aesklepieian model. After overcoming strong institutional resistance and unfounded rumors of misconduct, the program grew, moved to Powhatan Correctional Center in 1980, and lasted until late 1982, when it was closed after a decline in state revenues forced budget cuts and resignation of its director.

Thus, a number of prison-based therapeutic communities developed in the 1970s and through the early 1980s. A variety of models existed—Daytop, Aesklepieian, Phoenix House—but not all of the programs focused on drug abusers. Some were designed for sex offenders, some for disturbed inmates, and some for offenders with no particular disorder other than a history of criminal offending. The lifespan of the programs averaged five-to-seven years. Most closed when executive priorities changed and/or revenue shortfalls reduced funding availability. A few became corrupted when supervision weakened and contraband drugs were brought in to them. Some were never able to develop a true community. Others, like the twenty-year-old Stay'n Out program, remain viable today. In many cases, however, closed therapeutic communities were replaced by new therapeutic communities. It is important to note that the theoretical underpinnings and operating standards of therapeutic community practice for most of these early programs, except for the Stay'n Out program and Cornerstone, would have met few of today's therapeutic community standards.

The New Wave of Therapeutic Communites

The next new surge of prison-based therapeutic community, drug-abuse treatment programs—funded through the Federal Anti-Drug Abuse Act of 1986—were two major national technical assistance projects. The monies, in part, were granted on the success of the Stay'n Out program. During Projects REFORM (funded by the Bureau of Justice Assistance, 1984-87) and RECOVERY (funded by the Center for Substance Abuse Treatment, 1988-

91), the author and his colleague, Dr. Harry Wexler, along with a team of consultants, provided technical assistance to twenty-two states to initiate or expand comprehensive, statewide correctional drug treatment. These efforts had a catalytic effect on the correctional community.

As the REFORM project grew, other states, and even other nations, began seeking materials to guide the initiation of drug-abuse treatment programming for their correctional inmates. New service-delivery models were created that enhanced the continuity of treatment so that programming begun in the institution could continue after program participants were released. The Federal Bureau of Prisons' expansion of treatment is also an indirect beneficiary of these programs. In just 10 years, the Bureau of Prisons has gone from treating fewer than 4,200 inmates to the operation of 34 therapeutic communities, treating 30 percent of federal inmates with moderate-to-severe drug problems; those with less severe problems also receive services.

Project REFORM resulted in expanding, improving, and/or implementing 72 assessment and referral programs; 118 drug education programs; 71 drug resource centers; 82 in-prison 12-step programs; 15 urine monitoring programs; 128 prerelease counseling and referral programs; 49 postrelease treatment programs with parole or work release; and 77 modified therapeutic community, treatment programs.

In 1991, when funding for Project REFORM ended, a new national effort, Project RECOVERY, was funded by the Alcohol, Drug Abuse and Mental Health Administration to provide technical assistance and training services to demonstration prison drug-treatment programs and to continue the work begun by REFORM. Nine states participated along with the original group from REFORM, and the work continued for eighteen months. One net effect of these two projects was that by 1997, 110 therapeutic communities, as well as a variety of other programs, were operational in state and federal correctional institutions.

We noted earlier that $270 million was authorized over a five-year period beginning in 1996 for the RSAT block grant program, which provides funding for the development of substance-abuse treatment programs in state and local correctional facilities. Like REFORM, the RSAT program encourages states to adopt comprehensive approaches to substance-abuse treatment for offenders, including relapse prevention and aftercare services. In the less than two years since implementation of the act, already seventy programs have been started or enhanced in more than forty states. While not requiring that therapeutic community programs be established with these funds, the model treatment program criteria that are stipulated are based on the powerful findings of the therapeutic-community evaluation studies produced since the latter half of the 1980s.

Conclusion

Programs such as Stay'n Out cost about $3,000 per year, per inmate. The savings produced in reduced crime and drug use-associated costs alone, however, repay the cost of the treatment in two-to-three years. Moreover, the higher the investment in rehabilitating the most severe offender-addicts, the greater the probable impact. Substantial reductions in high-volume criminality have an immediate impact on the quality of life. Thus, with appropriate intervention applied for a sufficient duration, more than three out of four offenders are highly likely to reenter the community and lead socially acceptable lives. A great many of the successful graduates of these programs in the United States had long histories of serious property crime and violent crime; this finding has important implications for the use of this modality for other offenders.

The current research shows that therapeutic communities are effective with diverse locales and populations, and that even high-rate offenders can be helped dramatically. It is clear that the greater the investment in rehabilitating the most severe offender-addicts, the greater the probable impact. However, despite these positive signs, therapeutic communities are still limited in the number of offenders who can be given this opportunity, and by the number of trained persons available to deliver the treatment.

References

Belenko, S. and J. Peugh. 1998. *Behind Bars: Substance Abuse and America's Prison Population*. Technical Report. New York: National Center on Addiction and Substance Abuse at Columbia University.

De Leon, G. 1995. Therapeutic Communities for Addictions: A Theoretical Framework. *International Journal of the Addictions*. 30:1603-1645.

Field, G. 1984. The Cornerstone Program: A Client Outcome Study. *Federal Probation*. 48:50-55.

————. 1989. A Study of the Effects of Intensive Treatment on Reducing the Criminal Recidivism of Addicted Offenders. *Federal Probation*. 53:51-56.

————. 1992. Oregon Prison Drug Treatment Programs. In C. G. Leukefeld and F. Tims, eds. *Drug Abuse Treatment in Prisons and Jails*. NIDA Monograph No. 118. Washington, D.C: National Institute on Drug Abuse.

Inciardi, J. A. 1995. The Therapeutic Community: An Effective Model for Corrections-based Drug Abuse Treatment. In K. C. Haas and G. P. Alpert, eds. *The Dilemmas of Punishment*. Prospect Heights, Illinois: Waveland Press.

Inciardi, J. A., S. S. Martin, C. F. Butzin, R. M. Hooper, and L. D. Harrison. 1997. An Effective Model of Prison-based Treatment for Drug-involved Offenders. *Journal of Drug Issues*. 27:261- 278.

Lipton, D.S. 1995. The Effectiveness of Treatment for Drug Abusers under Criminal Justice Supervision. NIJ Research Report. Washington, D.C.: Department of Justice. November.

————. 1996. Prison-Based Therapeutic Communities: Their Success with Drug Abusing Offenders. *National Institute of Justice Journal*. 230: 12-20. February.

————. 1997. Drug Use Forecasting Data Trends: How We Can Use Them to Develop and Implement Programs in Corrections (and what we have to add). Paper presented at the National Correctional Conference, Washington, D.C., April 23, 1997.

————. 1998. Therapeutic Community Treatment Programming in Corrections. In Clive R. Hollin, ed. *London Handbook of Offender Assessment and Treatment*. London: John Wiley and Sons Ltd.

Martin, S. S., C. A. Butzin, and J. A. Inciardi. 1995. Assessment of a Multi-stage Therapeutic Community for Drug Involved Offenders. *Journal of Psychoactive Drugs*. 271:109-116.

Prendergast, Mohr, J. Wellisch, and G. P. Falkin. 1995. Assessment of and Services for Substance Abusing Women Offenders in the Community and Correctional Settings. *The Prison Journal*. 75(2), 240-256.

Wexler, H. K. 1995. The Success of Therapeutic Communities for Substance Abusers in American Prisons. *Journal of Psychoactive Drugs*. 27:3, 57-66.

Therapeutic Communities

Wexler, H. K., G. De Leon, G. Thomas, D. Kressel, and J. Peters. 1998. The Amity Prison TC Evaluation: Reincarceration Outcomes. *Criminal Justice and Behavior.*

Wexler, H. K., G. P. Falkin, and D. S. Lipton. 1988. A Model Prison Rehabilitation Program: An Evaluation of the "Stay'n Out" Therapeutic Community. Final Report to the National Institute on Drug Abuse, Rockville, Maryland.

———. 1990. Outcome Evaluation of a Prison Therapeutic Community for Substance Abuse Treatment. *Criminal Justice and Behavior.* 17:71-92.

~

Douglas S. Lipton, Ph.D., is a senior research fellow at the National Development and Research Institutes Inc. in New York.

Drug Courts and Jail-based Treatment:

Jail Setting Poses Unique Opportunity to Bridge Gap Between Courts and Treatment Services

By C. West Huddleston

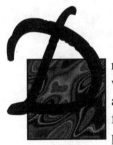

rug courts mark a turning back of the judicial clock to a time when judges were responsible for their own courts' operations; a defendant had to answer directly and immediately to a judge for his or her conduct; and a judge monitored each defendant's progress as his or her case moved slowly and purposefully through the judicial system.

The courts have been forced to move away from this level of personal involvement, largely because of an overwhelming workload, relying instead on an expedited case management model with segmented case management, sentencing guidelines, negotiated pleas, and other strategies.

The results have been mixed. While more cases are heard, each participant in a single defendant's case—court, probation, prosecution, and defense personnel—is responsible for only a small segment of the case. Often, dozens of judicial, probation, prosecution, and defense personnel see an offender over the course of a single case. No one has or is expected to take a larger view of the offender (or the system) because everyone has been given piecemeal authority.

What Are Drug Courts?

Drug courts differ significantly from previous attempts to manage and rehabilitate drug-using offenders. Rather than relying upon fragmented criminal justice and treatment systems, drug courts bring the full weight of all intervenors to bear, forcing the defendant to address his or her underlying substance abuse problem. The judge, prosecutor, defense counsel, substance-abuse treatment specialist, probation officer, law enforcement officer, correctional officer, educational and vocational experts, and community leaders create a unified system.

The drug court model typically entails:
- a single drug court judge and staff who provide leadership and focus
- expedited adjudication through early identification of appropriate program participants and referral to treatment as soon as possible after arrest
- intensive long-term treatment and aftercare for appropriate drug-using offenders
- comprehensive and well-coordinated supervision through regular status hearings before a single drug court judge to monitor treatment progress and program compliance
- increased defendant accountability through a series of graduated sanctions and rewards
- mandatory and frequent drug testing

The Judge's Role

The involvement of the judge is critical to the success of the drug court. According to Dr. Sally Satel, a psychiatrist and consultant to the Washington, D.C., drug court, the judge "serves as an authority figure . . . providing the attentive, dependable, if stern, parental approval that many addicts, coming from chaotic backgrounds and broken homes, seem to crave." The judge's active participation in the defendant's treatment begins at an inclusive "staffing" that generally occurs in the judge's chambers prior to a drug court hearing. During a staffing, representatives from probation, substance abuse treatment, case management, defense, and prosecution collaboratively update the drug court judge on a defendant's status. Armed with accurate and up-to-date information, the drug court judge then holds a status hearing, which occurs in open court. Here, the judge holds the defendant publicly accountable for his or her progress or lack thereof.

The drug court model allows the judge to use coercion to keep the defendant engaged in treatment. Leverage, coerced abstinence, and external pressure often are employed to keep the offender on track. "Addicts needn't want to change their lives, at least not at first, for a treatment program to succeed," Satel says. "With the fear of doing time hanging over his head, a drug abuser is more likely to stay and finish treatment. The longer he stays, the better his chances of turning his life around."

There is some evidence that without the coercive role of the judge, the impact of the drug court would be bleak. A recent survey reported that 80 percent of drug court participants indicated they would not have remained in the treatment program if they did not have to appear before a judge as part of the process.

Smart Punishment

In addition to the judge's active participation in the defendant's treatment, the drug court team relies on a pragmatic sentencing philosophy known as "smart punishment." Smart punishment is the imposition of the minimum amount of punishment necessary to achieve the twin sentencing goals of reduced criminality and drug usage. It relies on the use of progressive sanctions—the measured application of a spectrum of sanctions, whose intensity increases incrementally with the number and seriousness of program failures.

Like a carpenter who shows up at a job site with only a hammer, a judge who uses extended incarceration as the only sanction for substance abuse does not have the tools to get the job done. Indeed, the drug court judges have a variety of sentencing options at their disposal, including intensive supervision, counseling, educational services, residential treatment, medical interventions, drug testing, and program incentives, as well as incarceration.

In a drug court, progressive sanctions are applied in response to program failure or noncompliance, and incentives are granted incrementally, moving the offender steadily toward sobriety. There are immediate and direct consequences for all conduct. Sanctions follow violations and are applied as close to the time of failure as possible. Eventually, the sanctions themselves become an incentive for compliance.

Array of Programs

Although all drug courts have similar structures, not all drug courts are the same. The design and structure of drug court programs are developed at the local level, to reflect the unique strengths, circumstances, and capacities of each community. Many sectors of the community are integrally involved in the planning and implementation process of a drug court system, including the criminal justice system, substance-abuse treatment providers, law enforcement, and educational and community antidrug organizations.

Drug Courts and Jail-based Treatment

Columbia University's National Center on Addiction and Substance Abuse (CASA) has provided the first major academic review and analysis of drug court research to date. Steven Belenko of CASA reviewed thirty evaluations of twenty-four drug courts across the nation and concluded that a number of consistent findings emerge from available drug court evaluations. The CASA study is the first to look specifically at the effectiveness of the drug court model on offenders, comparing the drug court model to other forms of community supervision. The study found that drug courts provide closer, more comprehensive supervision and much more frequent drug testing and monitoring than some other forms of community supervision, such as probation and parole. More important, drug use and criminal behavior are substantially reduced while offenders are participating in drug court programs.

The CASA study further summarizes findings from the existing evaluations of both older and newer drug courts. Although the evaluations vary considerably in scope, methodology, and quality, the results are consistent in finding the following:

- Drug courts have been successful in engaging and retaining felony offenders in programmatic and treatment services who have substantial substance abuse and criminal histories but little prior treatment engagement.
- Drug courts provide more comprehensive and closer supervision of the drug-using offender than other forms of community supervision.
- Drug use and criminal behavior are substantially reduced while clients are participating in the drug court.
- Criminal behavior is lower after program participation, especially for graduates, although few studies have tracked recidivism for more than one year postprogram.
- Drug courts generate cost savings, at least in the short term, from reduced jail/prison use, reduced criminality, and lower criminal justice system costs.
- Drug courts have been successful in bridging the gap between the court and the treatment/public health systems and spurring greater cooperation among the various agencies and personnel within the criminal justice system, as well as between the criminal justice system and the community.

As drug courts have proven their effectiveness in controlling both the drug usage and criminality of drug-using offenders, communities successfully have expanded drug court programs to probationers, including drug-using offenders charged with nondrug offenses. American University's Drug Court Clearinghouse reports that 70 percent of drug courts now include probation-based or postplea programs and that the typical participant has at least a fifteen-year history of drug usage.

The Jail-based Treatment Gap

Although drug courts now are recognized as a successful criminal justice innovation, few jurisdictions to date have developed jail-based treatment programs that work successfully within the drug court framework.

According to the Bureau of Justice Statistics (Harlow, 1998), 11 million offenders pass through American jails each year, one-half to three-quarters testing positive for illicit drug use upon intake. More than half of jail inmates in 1996 were already under supervision at the time of their most recent arrest—almost one-third on probation, one-eighth on parole and one-eighth on bail or bond. Seven of ten jail inmates previously had been sentenced to probation or incarceration; more than 40 percent had served three or more sentences. Compared to jail inmates in 1989, inmates in 1996 reported a higher percentage of use of every type of drug except cocaine, with only 17 percent reporting prior participation in a treatment or self-help program.

In spite of scientific evidence that jail- and prison-based drug and alcohol programs can be effective in reducing recidivism, most jails have been slow to develop strong substance-abuse programs. A recent national survey noted that only 30 of 1,700 jails reported providing more than 10 hours of substance abuse treatment on average to inmates (Hughey and Klemke, 1996).

Jails offer a critical opportunity to meet offenders' substance-abuse problems early in the process. Jails are where individuals are screened, receive assessment, initial treatment services, social detoxification (stabilization), and where links to community treatment programs can take place.

In a review of criminal justice research, Carleton University researcher D. A. Andrews (1994) found that "there were no studies that found punishment alone reduced recidivism." If the goal is to close the revolving door by sustaining and spreading successful programs, then the next level for drug courts is to encourage the expansion of jail-based treatment programs, especially in those communities where drug courts exist.

Many drug courts depend on their local jails to either incarcerate defendants for a period of time prior to entering the drug court program or to house a defendant for a short period of time as a sanction for drug use. Since it is the objective of the drug court to keep the defendant engaged in treatment, treatment should be provided while the defendant provides a captive audience.

The challenge is to build on the documented success of drug courts and construct a bridge between county jails and existing drug courts, and provide effective jail-based treatment for drug court defendants wherever they are in the detainment process. We immediately must engage them in treatment services upon detainment and then refer them to outpatient and ancillary services, while providing supervision through the drug court program.

Several drug courts across the country have developed links with existing jail-based treatment programs. In New Haven, Connecticut, when a drug court defendant is ordered to serve jail time as a sanction for drug use, the judge asks the jail to give the defendant priority access to all counseling, Alcoholics Anonymous (AA), and Narcotics Anonymous (NA) programs that evening. In Denver, the drug court judge monitors defendants in both custody and non-correctional-therapeutic-community programs. In addition, a handful of drug courts have created comprehensive jail-based treatment programs that provide a continuum of care and accountability for drug court defendants.

San Bernardino, California

The San Bernardino County Sheriff's Department in San Bernardino, California, operates the Glen Helen Rehabilitation Center, a minimum-security residential treatment facility for jail inmates. The facility is aimed at drug-abusing offenders who have been classified carefully for minimum-security housing. Classification procedures are used to determine the risk that an inmate may pose while housed at the facility. Using information from the offender's criminal history, arrests, and drug and alcohol history, variables such as violence, stability, escape risk, gang affiliation, substance abuse, and current conviction are tallied via a point system to determine where the inmate will be housed. Once classified to the Glen Helen Rehabilitation Center, the inmate receives treatment and educational services, as well as job assignments, depending upon his or her needs.

The San Bernardino and Redlands drug courts have a unique relationship with the jail-based program. Jail staff are notified of the drug court referral by the court clerk. Drug court defendants then are placed into jobs within the facility that allow for attendance in all program groups and classes. Drug court defendants receive a multimodal approach to services at the Glen Helen Rehabilitation Center which includes substance-abuse counseling, Alcoholics Anonymous and Narcotics Anonymous support groups, anger management, parenting, life skills, basic education, literacy and GED classes, and a wide range of vocational classes.

After ten weeks of intensive treatment, the jail staff assesses each participant based on attitude, motivation, use of time, and tasks accomplished. These assessments are provided to the judge prior to status hearings. At that time, the drug court judge orders the defendant to continue treatment at the Glen Helen Rehabilitation Center, be released and referred to a community inpatient program, or be released and referred to outpatient services. In each case, the defendant remains in the drug court program, monitored by the judge. A 1995 impact evaluation of the San Bernardino program showed a significant reduction in recidivism of treated versus nontreated comparison groups.

Uinta County, Wyoming

The Uinta County drug court and the Uinta County Sheriff's Office have successfully implemented a jail-based treatment program for serious, repeat offenders or those who have failed at, or walked away from, other treatment programs. The jail-based treatment program is designed for a postsentence disposition where the defendant receives a six-month sentence and immediately enters the six-week, jail-based treatment program. While in the program, the defendant appears in drug court once a week for a status hearing. Once defendants complete the jail program, they appear in drug court for a sentence-reduction hearing and are referred to outpatient counseling and continued drug-court supervision through the five-phase system. Requirements gradually are reduced until defendants are graduated from the program.

A unique aspect of the Uinta County drug court program is that the jail-based treatment program personnel and the community aftercare treatment providers use the same systematic, offender-specific treatment modality, allowing for a true continuum of care. The jail administrator, as well as other jail personnel, are trained in the cognitive-behavioral treatment modality known as Moral Reconation Therapy (MRT®), which addresses the defendants' faulty decision-making, and helps them set and achieve goals. The results of the effort have been impressive, as recidivism has been reduced 30 percent, thus far.

Los Angeles County

In-custody drug treatment and drug-abuse resistance education programs in the Los Angeles County Jail provide a program bridge to the eleven adult drug courts in operation in the county. A drug court module for men has been set aside at the Century Regional Detention Facility, complete with space for meetings, acupuncture, and counseling. This module is isolated from the general population of the jail. A separate module for female inmates exists in a different facility. A private, licensed drug treatment provider operates the in-custody drug treatment programs.

A recently implemented drug court in Los Angeles County is the Sentenced Offender Drug Court. It requires completion of a mandatory, ninety-day, jail-based treatment phase in addition to any previous period of incarceration served as a condition of the initial grant of probation. The target population for this program includes probationers with severe drug addictions and repeated criminal justice system involvements. The purpose of the in-custody component is to accommodate incarcerative sentences, as well as to provide the first three months of treatment in a secure environment.

Unique to this in-custody program is the transitional housing made available to appropriate participants who do not have safe and sober living accommodations in the community. A preliminary cost-benefit analysis of the program has shown a savings to the county through use of the in-custody treatment program.

References

Andrews, D.A. 1994. An Overview of Treatment Effectiveness: Research and Clinical Principles. In *What Works: Bridging the Gap Between Research and Clinical Principles*. Longmont, Colorado: National Institute of Corrections.

Belenko, S. 1998. Research on Drug Courts: A Critical Review. *National Drug Court Institute Review*. I1:1-42.

Cooper, C. 1997. Drug Court Survey Report: Executive Summary. Washington, D.C.: Drug Court Clearinghouse and Technical Assistance Project, American University.

Field, G. 1989. The Effects of Intensive Treatment on Reducing the Criminal Recidivism of Addicted Offenders. *Federal Probation*. 534:51-56.

Harlow, C. W. 1998. Profile of Jail Inmates, 1996. Special Report Series NCJ 164620. Washington, D.C.: Bureau of Justice Statistics.

Hughey, R. and L. W. Klemke. 1996. Evaluation of a Jail-based Substance Abuse Treatment Program. *Federal Probation*. 604:40-44.

Lipton, D. S. 1996. Prison-based Therapeutic Communities: Their Success with Drug-abusing Offenders. *National Institute of Justice Journal*. 12-19.

Peters, R. H., W. D. Kerns, M. R. Murin, A. S. Dolente, and R. L. May. 1993. Examining the Effectiveness of In-jail Substance Abuse Treatment. *Journal of Offender Rehabilitation*. 193/4:1- 39.

Rouse, J. J. 1991. Evaluation Research on Prison-based Drug Treatment Programs and Some Policy Implications. *The International Journal of the Addictions*. 261:29-44.

Satel, S. 1998. Do Drug Courts Really Work? *City Journal*. 81-87.

U.S. General Accounting Office (GAO). 1997. *Drug Courts: Overview of Growth, Characteristics and Results*. Washington, D.C.: U.S. General Accounting Office.

Wexler, H. K., G. P. Falkin, and D. S. Lipton. 1990. Outcome Evaluation of Prison Therapeutic Communities for Substance Abuse Treatment. *Criminal Justice and Behavior*. 171:71-92.

Wexler, H. K., G. P. Falkin, D. S. Lipton, and A. B. Rosenblum. 1994. Progress in Prison Substance Abuse Treatment: A Five-year Report. *The Journal of Drug Issues*. 171:71-92.

≈

C. West Huddleston is deputy director of the National Drug Court Institute in Alexandria, Virginia. For further information on the programs described above, contact Mr. Huddleston at (703) 706-0576.

From the Institution to the Community:

Studies Show Benefits of Continuity of Care in Reduced Recidivism, Relapse Rates

By Gary Field, Ph.D.

*T*he effectiveness of jail and prison substance-abuse treatment has been well established over the years. Among inmate treatment programs, prerelease therapeutic communities (TC) have been the most studied, and have a well-documented record of success. For example, evaluations of New York's Stay'n Out therapeutic community examined the progress of more than 2,000 inmates during a ten-year period and found that the program was successful even with clients with extensive criminal records.

Studies also have shown that community-based offender drug treatment can be successful. Researchers Doug Anglin and his associates at the University of California at Los Angelos (Anglin and McGlothlin, 1984) present impressive long-term follow-up data on the California Civil Addict Program, a large-scale project involving programs across California that mandated long-term treatment for addicts in the 1960s and 1970s. More than forty independent evaluations also have been conducted of Treatment Alternatives to Street Crimes (TASC) programs, which identify, assess, and refer nonviolent offenders to treatment as an alternative or supplement to justice system sanctions. Studies of the TASC programs, which have been implemented throughout the country, have particular significance because they have focused on the transition of offenders from institutions to the community.

In short, there are institution prerelease models that work (for example, therapeutic communities), and there are community models that work (for example, intensive supervision with treatment). However, too little attention has been given to the process of transition from institution to community. Both criminal justice and substance-abuse treatment experts have observed that important gains made during incarceration are not being sustained when offenders return to the community because continuity of care is either inadequate or nonexistent.

According to University of South Florida researcher Roger Peters:

> Many offenders report feeling overwhelmed by the transition from a highly structured correctional environment to a less-structured environment following release. At this time of concentrated stress, an offender enters a culture where little or no support exists—no job, no money, weakened or broken family ties—with immediate needs to plan daily activities, to begin interacting constructively in nonadversarial relationships, and to manage personal or household finances and problems (Peters, 1993).

Authors in related fields of study have made similar observations. The juvenile justice field has been emphasizing the need for aftercare for several years. The recent and very intensive studies of boot camps and shock incarceration programs have begun to emphasize the critical component of aftercare in both theory and research (American Correctional Association, 1996, 1998).

Continuity of Treatment

Only very recently have researchers begun to examine the specific effects of continuity of offender treatment from institution to community on outcome-success rates. Jim Inciardi (1996) found that drug-involved offenders who participated in a continuum of drug treatment (prison-focused therapeutic-community-treatment followed by treatment in a work-release center) in the Delaware system had lower rates of drug use and recidivism than offenders in the institution program alone:

> The findings indicate that at eighteen months after release, drug offenders who received twelve-to-fifteen months of treatment in prison followed by an additional six months of drug treatment and job training were more than twice as likely to be drug-free as offenders who received prison-based treatment alone. Furthermore, offenders who received both forms of treatment were much more likely than offenders who received only prison-based

treatment to be arrest-free eighteen months after their release (71 percent compared to 48 percent).

In a similar study in California at the Donovan facility, researcher Harry Wexler (1996) found that drug-involved offenders who participated in both the Amity prison therapeutic-community program and the Amity community-based therapeutic community program upon release had substantially reduced rates of recidivism over those offenders who participated in the prison-based program alone. Wexler further presents a data comparison of California, Delaware, and Texas programs showing similar improved outcomes of prison treatment plus community treatment over prison treatment alone.

Oregon has taken a somewhat different approach. While the prison-based therapeutic community programs in Oregon always have stressed continuity of treatment, program planners hypothesized that shorter and less intensive prison programs with continuity of treatment in an intensive community program for inmates with lower levels of addiction and criminality would yield similar results to the more intensive therapeutic-community programs, which are targeted to more criminal and more highly addicted inmates. If this hypothesis is accurate, then even less-severely addicted inmates would be shown to benefit from continuity of services from institution to community.

In 1990, the Oregon Department of Corrections began a demonstration project to show the effects of a thorough transition program from institution to community treatment. Inmates began a three-to-six-month, prerelease day treatment program in an Oregon prison-release facility, then were followed intensively for six-to-nine months in community treatment and supervision.

Key program elements were as follows:

1. *Service providers "reach in" to the institution.* Parole and drug treatment services began while the individual was still incarcerated, usually several months before parole. Inmates from individual counties had their own groups led by county drug treatment providers.
2. *Joint institution/community-release planning.* Release center staff developed inmates' release plans cooperatively with the inmates, their parole officers, and drug treatment coordinators. Inmates were included in the planning process, and signed an agreement on program participation that

included a listing of graduated program incentives and sanctions.

3. *Intensive supervision.* Once the drug-involved offenders were paroled, they were placed under intensive supervision in the community.

4. *Continuity of treatment.* Group treatment continued into the community, usually with the same group leader and with many of the same members of the individual's institution group. Peer support for abstinence and recovery was an important theme of these groups.

5. *Careful management of incentives and sanctions.* Throughout the process, offenders were provided with incentives for program participation and sanctions for noncompliance or relapse. In the release center, participating inmates were given desirable housing, could earn extra pass time, were provided with special job skills counseling, and were given special consideration for release-subsidy funding. They were monitored more closely, and lost privileges according to a graduated schedule. In the community, program participants also were monitored more closely, experienced graduated sanctions, and were provided the incentives of housing, employment, and other specialized services.

Outcome studies of this program have shown that arrest rates of participating offenders dropped by 54 percent, and their conviction rates dropped by 65 percent during the year following treatment. In 1993, three more of these pre-release day treatment programs were added. The three programs vary in design and population served (one is for women with young children; one is for male Hispanics who primarily speak Spanish; one is rural), but each emphasizes preparation for community supervision and treatment. A recent study shows the effectiveness of these programs, including improvement in employment and community adjustment, along with decreases in recidivism and community burden.

Theoretical Underpinnings

The reasons for the importance of continuity of treatment from institution to community can be examined from the perspectives of the criminal justice system and the individual offender.

From the criminal justice system perspective, the offender is confronted with a system that really is not a system in the usual sense. Little program coordination exists between arrest, diversion, conviction, probation, revocation, jail, prison, and parole or postprison supervision. While there are examples of excellent coordination to be found between some of these points in the criminal justice system, they are exceptions.

Were an average person to examine a criminal justice flowchart and be asked where continuity would be the best, that person would probably identify the point of transfer from prison to community supervision. If the offender is under prison supervision and in a prison program, and is being sent to community supervision and a community program, what possible reason is there not to coordinate programs? Given that prison inmates include the most dangerous offenders in the criminal justice system, and given that heavy substance-abusing offenders are among the highest-risk offenders, and given that considerable societal resources are spent on prison supervision, prison treatment, community supervision, and community treatment, should not the public expect efficient and effective coordination of programs from institution to community supervision?

Offenders, particularly recidivistic offenders, frequently demonstrate antisocial characteristics. Part of antisocial behavior includes finding and exploiting any gap in supervision or monitoring. Therefore, the absence of continuity from institution to community programs can be expected to result in an undermining of treatment gains which, in turn, wastes treatment resources while decreasing community safety.

From the individual offender's perspective, leaving prison, particularly after a lengthy incarceration, can be an intimidating experience. Most people become overly comfortable with highly structured environments: a process called "institutionalization." Individuals with psychological disorders appear to have even more difficulty readjusting to community living after living in highly structured environments. This phenomenon seems to occur across disorders such as mental illness or addiction, although it may be expressed differently depending on the person and the disorder. Partly because of the disorder itself and partly because of anxiety surrounding the disorder, institutionalized individuals have difficulty transferring learning from one situation to another. What they learn in the institution program does not easily transfer to the community.

Institution programs start a recovery process in an environment in which structure helps the change process to begin, and which does not pose a risk to the community. But recovery and self-management skill-learning begun in the institution program need reinforcement and some degree of relearning in the community follow-up program. Without good coordination between programs, the offender's disorder, anxiety, or both are likely to weaken treatment gains and trigger a relapse. Parole officers have long observed the high-risk status of offenders newly released from prison. As has often been noted in the mental health treatment literature, rather than lament the institution-to-community transfer-of-learning problem exhibited by these individuals, the criminal justice system should program to account for it.

Obstacles to Continuity of Care

If continuity of offender treatment is necessary and shown to be effective, why is it still only the exception, rather than general practice? Several factors weigh against continuity practices. These impediments need to be identified clearly to overcome them and move forward.

1. *Segmentation of the criminal justice system.* The criminal justice system is not a discrete, well-coordinated system, but is actually a cluster of independent agencies and entities with separate justice responsibilities. These entities include jails, prisons, pretrial agencies, probation and parole agencies, the courts, law enforcement, and community organizations working with offenders. Successful transition of offenders into the community requires collaboration among all these entities. However, most of these agencies are under separate funding streams, with differing organizational missions, and they often have little understanding of the other components of the system.
2. *Lack of coordination between the criminal justice system and substance-abuse treatment programs.* Substance abuse treatment programs most often develop within health or human resource systems that have traditions, values, and goals that are different than the criminal justice system. Bringing these different perspectives together into a common mission can be challenging. Discontinuity occurs more frequently between community treatment and community supervision than it does between the institution treatment and the institution, but the community discontinuity often makes coordination between institution-treatment programs and community-treatment programs difficult.
3. *Loss of postrelease structure for offenders.* Those who have been incarcerated for extended periods of time may be lacking in many basic life skills and the ability to solve day-to-day problems. The decisions about these

new obligations can lead to serious consequences, yet often no individual or system is responsible for helping the offender prioritize and balance the challenges of life in the community.

4. *Loss of incentives and sanctions at release.* Formal incentives and sanctions to participate in treatment and to maintain prosocial behavior may not be as strong in the community as they are in the institution. Without these incentives to continue sobriety and a crime-free lifestyle, offenders struggling with community adjustment may slip into old patterns of behavior. This is particularly true when community supervision has been eliminated, or is not strongly enforced.

5. *Lack of services in the community.* There are a variety of services needed by the offender in transition. Many of these are considered "ancillary," although without them, treatment success is unlikely. For example, offenders will not be able to participate in outpatient treatment if they do not have housing and transportation. A range of services are necessary for effective treatment.

6. *Lack of treatment-provider experience with offenders.* In some areas, community substance-abuse treatment providers are inexperienced in adapting substance-abuse treatment to people with histories of criminal lifestyles. Lack of appreciation for the additional problems of criminal thinking and the anxieties surrounding release from incarceration significantly weaken community-based treatment. In a related problem, some community-treatment programs fail to recognize the work that has been done in the institution-treatment program, serving to further frustrate the offender and increase program dropouts.

7. *Community funding challenges.* The criminal justice population comprises a major percentage of those in need of substance-abuse treatment, yet within many community programs, there is a lack of specialized staff and few services targeted to meet offenders' needs. This is due in part to the fact that substance-abuse treatment agencies have not always identified offenders as a priority population, and agencies that provide community supervision do not always fund treatment services during probation or parole.

Successful Program Models

Strategies for offender-treatment continuity from institution to community can be organized conceptually into four types: outreach, reach-in, third-party, and mixed-program models.

In outreach programs, institution staff reach out to community supervision and treatment-program providers to ensure continuity. This model is most effective when case management resources are available within the institution, and when community services are not sufficiently organized to begin service before the offender leaves prison.

Reach-in programs are those where community supervision staff, treatment program staff, or both begin services before the offender leaves prison. This model requires an investment strategy approach by the community agency, which must recognize the advantage of anticipating problems rather than reacting to them after they occur. Oregon prison therapeutic community and prerelease day treatment programs have employed a number of strategies to build on this continuity of treatment model, including program design, interagency agreements, and funding that follows the inmate. To ensure continuity, Oregon's prison therapeutic communities directly fund the first two months of community treatment once the inmate is released from prison.

Third-party continuity means that an agency separate from corrections or treatment takes primary responsibility for ensuring service continuity. The third-party continuity programs are best-represented by TASC programs, which can be found in several jurisdictions across the country, including Alabama, Colorado, and Illinois. According to the TASC mission statement, TASC programs endeavor to address the justice system's concern for public safety while recognizing the need for community treatment to decrease substance abuse and thereby reduce criminal behavior. TASC participates in justice system processing as early as possible, identifying, assessing, and referring nonviolent offenders to treatment as an alternative or supplement to justice system sanctions. TASC then monitors the offenders' compliance with the expectations set for abstinence, employment, and social functioning.

The three program models noted above can be combined in mixed-continuity models. For example, the Amity program at the Donovan facility in California began as a prison therapeutic community, then developed its own follow-up, community-based therapeutic community for prison program graduates.

Conclusion

Research has shown the effectiveness of both institution and community substance-abuse treatment for offenders. However, too little attention has been given to the process of transition from institution to community. Recent studies demonstrate the added value of good coordination between institution and community supervision and treatment. Theoretical underpinnings and models of continuity of offender substance-abuse treatment from institution to community must be identified and replicated.

References

Altschuler, D. and T. Armstrong. 1996. Aftercare not Afterthought: Testing the IAP Model. *Juvenile Justice*. 3:15-22.

American Correctional Association. 1996. *Juvenile and Adult Boot Camps*. Lanham, Maryland.

———. 1998. "Shock Incarceration," in *Best Practices: Excellence in Corrections*. Lanham, Maryland: American Correctional Association.

Anglin, D. and W. McGlothlin. 1984. Outcome of Narcotic Addicted Treatment in California. In F. M. Tims and J. P. Ludford, eds. *Drug Abuse Treatment Evaluation: Strategies, Progress, and Prospects*. Research Monograph No. 51, Rockville, Maryland: National Institute on Drug Abuse.

Chaiken, M. 1989. *Prison Programs for Drug-involved Offenders*. Research in Action. Washington, D.C.: National Institute of Justice.

Cook, L. F. and B. Weinman. 1988. Treatment Alternatives to Street Crime. In C. G. Leukefeld and F. M. Tims, eds. *Compulsory Treatment of Drug Abuse: Research and Clinical Practice*. Research Monograph No. 86. Rockville, Maryland: National Institute on Drug Abuse.

DeLeon, G. 1984. Program-based Evaluation Research in Therapeutic Communities. In F. M. Tims and J. P. Ludford, eds. *Drug Abuse Treatment Evaluation: Strategies, Progress and Prospects*. Research Monograph No. 51. Rockville, Maryland: National Institute on Drug Abuse.

Field, G. 1989. The Effects of Intensive Treatment on Reducing the Criminal Recidivism of Addicted Offenders. *Federal Probation*. 53:51-56.

Field, G. and M. Karecki. 1992. Outcome Study of the Parole Transition Release Project. Salem, Oregon: Oregon Department of Corrections.

Finigan, M. 1997. Evaluation of Three Oregon Pre-release Day Treatment Substance Abuse Programs for Inmates. Washington, D.C.: Center for Substance Abuse Treatment.

Hubbard, R. L., J. V. Rachal, S. G. Craddock, and E. R. Cavanaugh. 1984. Treatment Outcome Prospective Study (Tops): Client Characteristics and Behaviors, Before, During and after Treatment. In F. M. Tims and J. P. Ludford, eds. *Drug Abuse Treatment Evaluation: Strategies, Progress and Prospects*. Research Monograph No. 51. Rockville, Maryland: National Institute on Drug Abuse.

Inciardi, J. A. 1996. *A Corrections-based Continuum of Effective Drug Abuse Treatment*. Washington, D.C.: National Institute of Justice.

Leshner, A. 1997. Addiction is a Brain Disease, and it Matters. *Science*. 278:45-46.

Leukefeld, C. G. and F. M. Tims. 1988. *Compulsory Treatment of Drug Abuse: Research and Clinical Practice*. Research Monograph No. 86. Rockville, Maryland: National Institute on Drug Abuse.

Lipton, D. 1995. *The Effectiveness of Treatment of Drug Abusers Under Criminal Justice Supervision*. Washington, D.C.: National Institute of Justice.

MacKenzie, D. and E. Hebert. 1996. *Correctional Boot Camps: A Tough Intermediate Sanction*. Washington, D.C.: National Institute of Justice.

MacKenzie, D. and C. Souryal. 1994. *Multisite Evaluation of Shock Incarceration*. Washington, D.C.: National Institute of Justice.

National Task Force on Correctional Substance Abuse Strategies. 1991. *Intervening with Substance-abusing Offenders: A Framework for Action*. Washington, D.C.: National Institute of Corrections.

Peters, R. H. 1993. Relapse Prevention Approaches in the Criminal Justice System. In T. T. Gorski, J. M. Kelley, L. Havens, and R. H. Peters, eds. *Relapse Prevention and the Substance-abusing Criminal Offender*. Technical Assistance Publication (TAP) Series, Number 8. Rockville, Maryland: Center For Substance Abuse Treatment.

Petersilia, J., S. Turners, and E. Deschences. 1992. The Costs and Effects of Intensive Supervision for Drug Offenders. *Federal Probation.* 4:12-170.

Simpson, D. 1984. National Treatment System Based on the Drug Abuse Program (DARP) Follow-up Research. In F. M. Tims and J. P. Ludford, eds. *Drug Abuse Treatment Evaluation: Strategies, Progress and Prospects.* Research Monograph No. 51. Rockville, Maryland: National Institute on Drug Abuse.

Weinman, B. A. 1992. *Coordinated Approach for Drug-abusing Offenders: TASC and Parole.* Research Monograph No. 118. Rockville, Maryland: National Institute on Drug Abuse.

Wexler, H., G. Falkin, and D. Lipton. 1988. *A Model Prison Rehabilitation Program: An Evaluation of the Stay 'n Out Therapeutic Community.* A Final Report to the National Institute on Drug Abuse by Narcotic and Drug Research, Inc.

Wexler, H. 1996. The Amity Prison TC Evaluation: Inmate Profiles and Reincarceration Outcomes. Prentation for the California Department of Corrections.

~

Gary Field, Ph.D., is administrator of counseling and treatment services for the Correctional Programs Division of the Oregon Department of Corrections. This report was prepared at the request of the Office of National Drug Control Policy and presented at a conference hosted by the Office of National Drug Control Policy in March, 1988. Some of the ideas presented in this paper are more thoroughly discussed by the author and others in the Center for Substance Abuse Treatment publication, Continuity of Offender Treatment from Institution to the Community. *Rockville, Maryland (In press).*

Corrections' Voice in America's Drug Problem

By General Barry R. McCaffrey (Retired)*

I am honored to do the job that I am doing now. I take great pride in being part of the group of Americans—men and women—in the federal government, state and local government, and more important, in law enforcement, in corrections, treatment facilities, drug education programs: educators, counterdrug coalitions, and parents who are involved in trying to manage this incredible problem in America.

In the time I have been involved in this effort, I have been tutored by some incredibly aware and experienced people who have insights, models, and experience. But if there is one voice that has not been at the table, it is the voice of the corrections community. We are going to have to correct that. I have asked your ACA executive director and your president to make me a part of their thinking. I have asked them to take part in discussing this national issue. And, we clearly have to take into account what you are facing.

The first thing we have to recognize is that most Americans do not use drugs and do not abuse alcohol. Thank God, in today's America, most of us do not even smoke cigarettes. There are 265 million of us, and we are one of the most hard-working groups on the face of the earth. We join associations. We pay our taxes. We have the highest church-going rate of any western nation except the Irish.

We are a pretty remarkable lot of people, but unfortunately, 12 million out of 265 million of us are using illegal drugs regularly. This has produced a small percentage—3.6 million—who are addicted to illegal drugs. If you look at that 3.6 million, there is an even smaller percentage of about 2.7 million people who are chronic, hard-core addicts. This group of 2.7 million people is at the heart and soul of many of the enormous challenges facing America today.

Drugs are a source of a considerable amount of AIDS in America, industrial accidents, absenteeism, teenage pregnancy, spousal abuse, violence, and property crimes. All of these are driven partially or principally by the use of illegal drugs. It is a tragedy in America. And the numbers are so gigantic, it is hard to make much sense out of them. I myself wear a little gold memory bracelet with the name "Tish Elizabeth Smith" on it to remind myself of this perfect girl who died last year in her first semester at university smoking heroin and crack cocaine. Her mother pulled the plug at the end of seven days, and away she went to become one of the 20,000 dead who were caught up in this problem. I do not need to tell you about it. You are looking at the end results of drug abuse in America.

Now, here is a problem for us. We have the unenviable position of having put 1.6 million Americans behind bars at local, state, and federal levels. We have the highest per capita rate of incarceration of any nation on the face of the earth. I would say a third of those in the state systems are there for drug-related reasons. And two-thirds of those in the federal system are there for drug-related reasons.

I am absolutely persuaded that if we are to solve the drug problem in America, drugs have to remain socially disapproved and against the law, and the police must uphold the law. If we do not do that, most of us believe that education and prevention programs and drug treatment programs simply will not work.

Sometimes I am asked if I object to the fact that we have spent an enormous amount of resources on fighting drug abuse and still have seen the federal prison population skyrocket 311 percent and the state system 237 percent. Do I object to the fact that we have gone from spending $3.1 billion in corrections in 1980 up to $17.7 billion in 1994? Do I object to the fact that drug offenders account for such an enormous part of the population? No, I do not. However, I do object to the fact that we spend a little over $3 a head per child in America on drug education and prevention. And I bitterly object to the fact that we have about half the treatment capacity in America that we need for these 3.6 million addicted Americans. In the prison system, we have a tiny fraction of the capability we need.

So, we have 2.7 million chronic, hard-core addicts consuming two-thirds of all the drugs in America. We say it is 240 metric tons of cocaine and 10 metric tons of heroin. Two-thirds of it is consumed by that population, and 80 percent of them are involved, in a given year, in the criminal justice system. You in corrections are going to see them. You simply cannot abuse alcohol and marijuana, cocaine and crack, or dangerous drugs such as methamphetamine, and not end up in the criminal justice system. But have we given you the adequate tools to do your jobs?

If you and I go out and randomly grab an experienced narcotics officer, an experienced sheriff, or a police chief and say, "What are we doing right now to deal with this problem? Does it make sense?" The answer is, "No, of course it doesn't." We have failed to convince city councils, state legislatures, and the U.S. Congress that drug treatment programs are a good option for the taxpayer. It is cheaper for you to provide treatment than it is to lock them up. It is clearly cheaper for you to do this than to tolerate somewhere between 300 and 900 felonies a year for heroin addicts. There are not many of them in our society. We say there are 600,000 heroin addicts in America, but they are out there stealing probably $1,000 a day of stuff from our neighborhoods to sell to maintain their heroin habit at $250 a day. It simply does not make sense to not understand that this chronic relapsing disorder does respond to effective drug treatment with follow-on care in the community. We have got to make that case.

The other thing we must make the case for is that it is appropriate that Americans are sick to death of the violent crime and the depravity and spiritual and moral failure that come along with extensive drug abuse. People do not use drugs because they are morally depraved. They use drugs because they are fun. They give intense pleasure. Who needs friends when you have heroin? When we look at our fellow employees or one of our own children using heroin, it is disgusting. You act like a jerk when you are using drugs. You are nauseated. Your skin crawls. You are constipated. You have lost your sex drive. That is the good news. The bad news is that then you get addicted. As experienced police officers will tell you, there are some people who like being criminals, but nobody likes being addicted. It is a life of unending misery.

Corrections' Voice in America's Drug Problem

That is what we are giving you to safeguard, rehabilitate, and send back to America. Yet, we are not giving you the tools to do that. We are going to have to solve it. We are going to have to have a different debate and a different dialog. We are going to have to understand that while being tough on crime is essential, we do not need to tolerate drug abuse in our workplace, our homes, or our schools. At the same time, we must sort out who we are putting in prison and why. We have to give the drug court system the flexibility to do things like break the cycle. You either get jailed, take treatment, or both. There is an intelligent decision maker—a judge or an official—who makes these calls and who will follow you for a year or more. The time to start worrying about drug abuse is not with a nineteen-year-old male felon. The time to start worrying about drug abuse in America is the sixth grade, which is where we see the onset of serious drug exposure in our society. Drug use among children has doubled in the last five years. Among eighth-graders, it is up three-fold. We are going to see a wave of violence and crime and pain ten years down the line the likes of which we have not seen since the early 1970s if we do not get organized and address this problem.

Children are at risk. Where are teenagers between 3 P.M. and 7 P.M.? We simply have to offer options like boys and girls clubs, sports programs, junior ROTC, and other activities to keep youth engaged, or clearly they will respond to the tutor they have, which is the television set. We look at our children when they finish high school, and they have spent 12,000 hours in formal classroom instruction. But, they have watched 15,000 hours of television. Kids do not have problems. We have problems. We have to get better organized in dealing with our sons and daughters.

When it comes to the prison system, whether it is federal, state, or local, we are testing the notion of breaking the cycle. You either can do time, do drug treatment, or both. We need integrated drug testing systems. We need court-authorized graduated sanctions. We need treatment programs, residential, in the system, and follow-on. We need offender tracking and rehabilitation. We cannot get money out of Congress and state legislatures if we cannot explain what we did with it. Finally, we must pay for aftercare and probably a drug court system to be in charge of that problem. If you do not have aftercare, you do not have a drug treatment program.

We also are learning more as we study these issues. We are getting a notion that if you are using pot and alcohol as a twelve-year-old, you are setting yourself to rewire the neurochemical function of your brain. You are going to end up as a different person. It is not a moral weakness now. It is not a failing. It is not a compulsion. Your brain is working differently.

I normally try to remind audiences that three out of four people abusing drugs are employed. One of the highest rates of drug addiction or alcohol addiction in America is among anesthesiologists and doctors who prescribe medicines. When they end up addicted in their forties to Percodan and end up in the Talbot Marsh Clinic in Atlanta at a several-thousand-dollar program, the neurochemical process that they are trying to fight is the same as a nineteen-year-old lad in Los Angeles or a fourteen-year-old girl in Rhode Island.

Drug addiction in America is not somebody else's problem. It is not an urban problem. It is not a poor people's problem. It is not a minority problem. It is all of our problem, and I do not need to tell you that, because you end up with that problem, and you are supposed to take care of it and make it better and send each one back to a productive life in society. Let me, if I may, tell you straight out that I am enormously proud of what you people do, what you stand for, and the absolutely awesome professionalism you bring to bear in the task.

∼

General Barry R. McCaffrey (Ret.) is the director of the Office of National Drug Control Policy in Washington, D.C.

*This is an edited version of the speech that General McCaffrey gave at the American Correctional Association's Winter Conference in Indianapolis, Indiana on January 28, 1997.

Hot New Technologies

By Gabrielle deGroot

*I*n 1993, prison administrators in California heard rumors of an impending inmate outbreak. The word was out that a handful of inmates had built a tunnel underneath the Lompoc Federal Correctional Institution, and were planning to make a break for freedom. Special Technologies Laboratories (STL) was called in to investigate. A team from the Santa Barbara-based company arrived on the scene the next day with equipment in hand, and using a new technology called ground penetrating radar (GPR), were able to locate the elusive tunnel, as well as several other escape routes used by inmates in the past.

Ground penetrating radar works much the way the old Geiger counters did, held in the hand and swept across the ground by an operator. Only instead of detecting metal, the ground-penetrating radar system detects changes in ground composition, including voids, such as those created by a tunnel. If it sounds a bit like science fiction, that may be because it is—at least, in part. Officials at Lompoc did not really have an imminent outbreak at hand. Instead, they had invited Special Technologies Laboratories to the facility to test out their new pulsed radar technology. And it worked well, demonstrating that ground-penetrating radar could be used in a real-life scenario should the occasion ever arise.

In fact, ground-penetrating radar is just one of many hot new technologies being deployed or tested in the corrections field today. Satellite monitoring, heartbeat monitoring, body cavity scanning, the using of smart cards—these are just a few of the applications of the cutting-edge technology under development.

"Ten years ago, there were very few companies that specialized in technology for prisons. We were the forgotten industry," says Larry Cothran, executive officer of the California Department of Corrections' Technology Transfer Committee. "But then the Cold War ended, and all of a sudden, you had a lot of companies trying to convert their military hardware to corrections and law enforcement." Today, many of these technologies are coming to market—technologies that can save taxpayers millions and improve the safety of inmates and officers.

Perimeter Fencing

Back in 1992, California began installing the first electric fences around its prisons. The fences are lethal, killing anything and anyone who comes into contact with them. At the time, skeptical industry observers said the system would never work, and never would be widely accepted in the field. Today, all of California's thirty-three prisons are surrounded by electric fencing, and six other states are planning to install them.

The reason is simple: electric perimeter fences work extraordinarily well. Not only has no one escaped over the fences since they were installed in California, but the fences eliminate the need for twenty-four-hour watchtower surveillance, saving countless personnel hours. "When you take the men out of the towers, that's five positions per tower and about twelve towers per prison. You can see this is a tremendous savings," Cothran says. "We estimate that we're saving taxpayers $32 million per year, about $1 million per prison."

Heartbeat Monitoring

The weakest security link in any prison has always been the sallyport, where trucks unload their supplies and where trash and laundry is taken out of the facility. Over the years, inmates have hidden in loads of trash, old produce, laundry—any possible container that might be exiting the facility. Today, a company run by former Texas Governor Mark White is marketing a new technology that can detect the heartbeat of a person hidden in a vehicle. The Advanced Vehicle Interrogation and Notification System (AVIAN) being marketed by Geo Vox Security works by identifying the shock wave generated by the beating heart, which couples to any surface the body touches.

"Regardless of the size of the vehicle, if a person is in it, it is moving to the tune of that person's heartbeat," explains Leo LeBaj, program manager of the National Security Program Office at Oakridge National Laboratory, where the system was developed. "The system takes all the frequencies of movement, such as the expansion and contraction of the engine, and rain hitting the roof, and determines if there is a pattern similar to a human heartbeat."

According to the AVIAN website (http://www.beicomm.com/avian), a potential escapee can be identified in less than two minutes after two specialized AVIAN sensors are placed on the vehicle. Prisons can buy the system for $50,000, or lease it for $1,000 per month. If this seems high, LeBaj notes that the average cost of locating and capturing an escaped inmate is estimated at $750,000.

Satellite Monitoring

It is relatively easy to keep track of offenders when they are behind bars, but correctional officers always have had difficulty monitoring offenders placed on home detention, especially those barred from contacting their victims. That is because electronic monitoring works only insofar as the offender follows the rules, reporting in at the designated times and giving the computer the correct codes when called. If an offender leaves home unexpectedly, his or her ankle bracelet will sound an alarm, but law enforcement officers often have no further way of tracking the offender. Until now. Pro Tech Monitoring Inc. of Palm Harbor, Florida, has developed a system to monitor offenders by satellite using cellular technology combined with the federal government's global positioning system of satellites. As with the regular electronic monitoring system, each offender wears an ankle bracelet, but he or she also carries a three-pound portable tracking device (smart box), programmed with information on his or her geographical restrictions.

For instance, a sex offender may be forbidden to come within five miles of his victim's home or workplace, or a pedophile may be barred from getting close to a school. A satellite monitors the geographic movements of the offender, either in real time or by transmitting the information to the smart box, for later retrieval. If an offender violates his or her boundaries, the information can be transmitted directly to the police, along with the offender's geographic location. The smart box and the ankle bracelet also squawk loudly when boundaries are breached, alerting potential victims.

"This will put teeth in a judgment, particularly for sex offenders and pedophiles," says Bob Martinez, former Florida governor and president of Pro Tech. Already, the system is being tested in Lackawanna County, Pennsylvania, for domestic violence and sex offender cases. In addition, the Florida Department of Corrections earlier this year awarded Pro Tech a five-year contract to use the system in Florida. The cost of the program runs from the mid-teens to the low-20s per offender per day. Martinez points out that this cost is still far lower than keeping the offender behind bars.

Smart Cards

If there is anything that correctional administrators hate most, it is the paper-work that goes along with keeping track of each inmate. Every time an inmate receives an aspirin for a headache, or buys toothpaste from the commissary, a prison clerk must record the transaction and file it away.

Now comes the smart card, a plastic card embedded with a computer chip that will store all types of information about an inmate: his or her movements, medical care, commissary purchases, treatment needs, meals eaten—any information at all that pertains to the inmate. Smart card developer Battelle Inc., of Columbus, Ohio, plans to test the technology at the Ohio Women's Reformatory in Marion later this year, as part of a grant from the National Institute of Justice, says Steve Morrison, program manager and deputy direc-tor of corrections for the National Law Enforcement and Corrections Technology Center in Charleston, South Carolina. "This is one of the biggest new innovations in corrections technology today," Morrison says. "When it's implemented, this will really reduce the paperwork in prisons—the paper-work and the manpower."

More to Come

Still other hot new technologies under development include:
- X-ray body scanners, which test for concealed weapons and contraband hidden in body cavities
- Noninvasive drug testing, using eye scans and patches placed on the skin
- A smart gun, which is computer coded so it cannot be fired by anyone other than the registered user (this technology, under development by

Sandia Labs, links the gun's trigger mechanism to a bracelet or ring worn by the officer)

- A language translator, for use by law enforcement and correctional officers to communicate with nonnative inmates
- Walk-through metal detectors that can pinpoint exactly where the metal is

The development of corrections-specific technology is proceeding at breakneck pace, with new technologies coming online every few months. And as companies compete for corrections business, the cost of the new technology will continue to decline, even as the technology improves. That is good news for corrections.

"The costs are starting to go down," Morrison says. "With the downsizing of the U.S. government, everyone is looking at law enforcement and corrections as the golden goose."

∽

Gabrielle deGroot is the former managing editor of Corrections Today *magazine.*

Internet Use and Access

By Earl Kellow and Joseph Clark

In the fall of 1995, the Florida Department of Corrections was faced with a dilemma. The internet was becoming immensely popular and was growing exponentially in the number of sites, quantity of information, and ease of use. Increasingly, staff within the department were asking for access to the internet and requesting permission to establish internet e-mail accounts for work use. Yet, the department had no existing internet use policy. There was no overall plan for embracing this "hot" new technology, nor were there any procedures or guidelines in place for staff to follow. Complicating the issue was the fact that there was—and still is—a lot of hype, misinformation, and ignorance concerning the internet.

Burning Issues

Sorting out the reality of the internet from the marketing hype presented a challenging task, but the Florida Department of Corrections was not about to ignore such a potentially rich source of information and research, nor such a readily available public relations and internal communications tool. The department's information technology section began by researching and drafting a formal internet policy document. This document answered several basic questions:

- Is there a benefit to be gained by department staff accessing the internet?
- If so, which staff should be allowed access?
- What authority within the department's organization structure should be designated to grant employees' access requests?
- What is the proper use of the internet by department employees?
- How should staff be advised on proper internet etiquette?

- How can the department protect itself from lawsuits or embarrassing situations resulting from staff use?
- What responsibilities does an employee assume when granted access to the internet?
- How does department management ensure that employees are using the internet properly and not abusing the privilege?
- Within the organization, what office/unit/committee is charged with setting internet-related standards and serving as the focal point for internet issues?
- What financial impact, if any, is associated with internet use by employees?
- Should inmates be allowed access to the internet in any manner?

The policy document was researched, drafted, and circulated for comment before being formally adopted in December 1995.

Lessons Learned

The department has provided employee access to the internet for almost eighteen months and has made the following observations:

- Early on, the department decided not to allow inmates direct access to the internet. Time has proven this to be a good policy decision.
- Access to the internet has benefited staff and the department, as they tap into the vast resources of the internet as a research and communications tool.
- Most staff have exercised good judgment and have not abused the access privilege. They have not wasted a lot of time "surfing" the internet and have exercised good internet etiquette.
- There have been no embarrassing internet-related incidents. The spirit of the policy has been followed.

The authority for granting access was pushed to the lowest level possible. Recognizing that only immediate supervisors really knew what potential use an employee may make of the internet, the department made the employee and his or her immediate supervisor responsible for proper use. Managers were asked to oversee their various sections, offices, or areas of responsibility for compliance with the department's internet policies and procedures. So far, this seems to have worked well. Any financial charges resulting from use of the internet also are handled by the work unit incurring these charges.

The department has received many positive comments regarding the new website—both from the public and from department of corrections employees. An important function of the site has been to get the "corrections story" out to the public. It serves as an ideal medium to tell the "other" side of issues that may have been presented in a less-than-positive light by the news media. For example, one of the most visible links refutes "Eight Common Misconceptions" about inmates and corrections—such as the belief that inmates never work—and backs up its arguments with facts and figures. Additionally, breaking news and press releases can be posted on the site in a timely fashion.

The internet also is beginning to be used to reach remote sites of the department. Any site with a personal computer and either a dial-up or a direct connection to the internet now can participate in the more up-to-date capabilities of local area network (LAN) systems. This is being used for e-mail, sending attachments and documents, and basic office automation functions.

What is New?

In the near future, the department will deploy its own internet server to permit greater autonomy and customization of our web presence. An intranet server capability also is in the works. Both projects will require department staff to assume the responsibility for implementing both servers, installing firewalls, and generally engaging in the ongoing support role of internet content provider. This will require dedicated resources, but the payoff will be worth the investment. The intranet server—distributing up-to-the-minute information targeted at department of corrections staff—will serve to increase communications both internally and externally.

Recent developments within the agency have prompted some minor modifications of the publishing process for the department's website, and thus changes to the internet policy and procedure document. The Florida Department of Corrections has appointed a full-time webmaster and has established an internet editorial committee, which reviews all requests for items to be added to the department's website and any policy changes under consideration. This committee keeps tabs on the changing internet world and updates the internet policy accordingly. The webmaster serves as the focal point for all the information flowing to the department's official website and advises the department on changing needs, issues, and capabilities on the worldwide web.

What to Say

If your agency is ready to create a website of its own, you will need to move from the role of internet receiver/consumer to that of information source/producer. These guidelines will help you make the transition.

How do you determine what to put on your website? First, do not reinvent the wheel. Your agency already has hundreds of pages of documents that are perfect for a website: reports, brochures, press releases, and so forth. You already have made the sometimes difficult decisions about whether or not to release these documents to the public—they are out there already. All you need to do is convert them into the proper format for the web, and today's print-production software (word processing, desktop publishing, and so on) has a number of features to make the conversion easier than it was just a few months ago. Choose existing public documents that reinforce the message or theme you are trying to get across: reducing misconceptions, justifying additional budget requests, enhancing the agency's image, and other standard public relations strategies. Your agency probably already has a communications officer who can make these decisions.

Kill two birds with one website. Consider adding information that not only will support the communications goals outlined above, but also will cut down on staff workload. How many hours are spent answering requests for information? How often is this information inconsistent? Put frequently requested documents and other information on your site. Most journalists have web access and will be glad to know they can visit the site at any time. If you can provide timely access to inmate data online (via a database front-end), think of the calls it might reduce!

Try to eliminate "dead tree" thinking. Do not limit your site to what can be printed on paper. The web is movies! Sound! Animation! For example, the Department of Corrections added a Java applet that shows a "time-lapse" view of prison construction, as well as a VRML (3-D) depiction of a prison cell that visitors can zoom in on and rotate to any viewing angle. Neither of these is possible on paper. Remember, however, that multimedia comes with a price tag. Files are generally rather large and therefore download times are longer. It may be difficult for some visitors to access some of the more cutting-edge multimedia. For this reason, choose your content with care.

Create an editorial board and solicit staff ideas. Some of your best ideas will come from staff who have no connection to the web effort. As with most other organizational activities, you must encourage bottom-up participation to enhance quality. Your more savvy users may not be in MIS or communications departments. An editorial board helps your web management staff ensure that all sectors of the agency are represented, and can help you spot potentially troublesome messages before they are delivered to the outside world. Without adding horrendous overhead, you can set up a submission approval process that ensures careful consideration of items while encouraging speedy publication and updating.

Fresher is better—but not always. The ubiquitous "under construction" sign on websites reflects the constant change going on there. Imagine a gigantic library in which nearly all the books are revised and updated on a weekly, or even daily, basis. How dusty and archaic a book from last year would seem! Websites, too, must remain current, and you should make sure your information is not "stale." On the other hand, information with a long "shelf life" can be a good candidate for inclusion on a website, especially if you can make it dynamic or interesting. Inmate narratives, historical photographs, and other content should be considered.

Above all, be personal, professional, and local. Consider using the website to promote specific accomplishments of star employees, thereby showcasing the professionalism of your staff. Finally, encourage reciprocal links between pages devoted to local institutions/offices and "hometown" websites to show your role in the community.

~

Earl Kellow (kellow.earl@mail.dc.state.fl.us) is chief information officer for the Florida Department of Corrections. Joseph Clark is the department of correction's former webmaster.

The Internet as a Technology and Information Resource:

The Corrections Practitioner's Guide to 'Surfing the Net'

By David Hart and Garry Pate

The boss has asked you to research information on a certain technology your facility wants to purchase. Conventional wisdom tells you to use the resources with which you are most comfortable, such as contacting a colleague or another facility to see exactly what they have been using or which product they recommend. Next, you might try looking in the phonebook or an old American Correctional Association conference program for a listing of manufacturers. You also might rely on word-of-mouth or a company's reputation. In the past, all of these resources would have given you a starting point, but times have changed. Today, corrections practitioners have a faster, and more reliable, resource—the internet.

The same internet that is helping your children learn more efficiently and providing you with up-to-the-minute sports scores, weather, and news also can help corrections practitioners learn about technology. On the internet, criminal justice practitioners have access to government and business websites addressing new products, services, and technologies. However, pinpointing the information you need can be either a pleasant journey or a trying experience. One of the secrets of traveling this tangled and extensive information highway is knowing where to begin.

Government Agencies

Your starting point on the internet might be those federal agencies with websites. The federal government maintains a number of websites that offer a variety of information about correctional programs, products, and technologies. The U.S. Department of Justice maintains a website at http://

www.usdoj.gov/. As you scroll through the introduction, you are offered two choices: to search the Justice Department's web servers, or to search the Department of Justice and all federal government servers. Choose the second option; then, at the next prompt, type in "corrections technology." This search will result in more than 7,000 documents relating to grant information, technology, jobs, and studies. From this website, you also will find links to:

- The Federal Bureau of Prisons (BOP) at http://www.bop.gov
- The National Institute of Corrections (NIC) at http://www.bop.gov/nicpg/nicmain.html

Both of these sites offer a variety of information concerning programs and services provided by the Bureau of Prisons.

Another excellent resource is the website of the Department of Justice's Office of Justice Programs (OJP) at http://www.ojp.usdoj.gov/. The Office of Justice Programs' mission is to provide federal leadership in developing the nation's capacity to prevent and control crime, administer justice, and assist crime victims. From Office of Justice main page, you can link to:

- The Bureau of Justice Assistance at http://www.ojp.usdoj.gov/BJA/, which provides comprehensive information on funding, evaluation, training, technical assistance, and information about state and community criminal justice programs
- The Bureau of Justice Statistics at http:// www.ojp.usdoj.gov/bjs/, which provides criminal justice statistics

The National Institute of Justice (NIJ), at http://www.ojp.usdoj.gov/nij/, is the research and development branch of the Department of Justice and provides many links to programs and services. Two popular National Institute of Justice programs are its National Criminal Justice Reference Service (NCJRS) and its National Law Enforcement and Corrections Technology Center (NLECTC).

- NCJRS, at http://www.ncjrs.org/, has one of the most comprehensive online sources of criminal and juvenile justice information in the world. NCJRS provides full text and abstracts of thousands of criminal justice-related publications on its website.
- NLECTC, at http://www.nlectc.org, is a program of the National Institute of Justice's Office of Science and Technology and offers an online gateway to law enforcement and corrections technology through its website—JUSTNET. JUSTNET provides information on new

technologies, equipment, and other products and services available to the law enforcement, corrections, and criminal justice communities, including access to a searchable database of more than 4,000 available products and technologies.

Specific Technologies

JUSTNET also provides information on projects funded by the National Institute of Justice, including:

- *Radar-Based, Through-the-Wall Surveillance Systems*: The National Institute of Justice, through a Joint Department of Justice/Department of Defense Program Steering Group , is sponsoring the development of a portable, through-the-wall surveillance device developed by the Raytheon Co. It employs radar that can locate and track an individual through concrete or brick walls, and also measures and displays the distance to that individual. The National Institute of Justice plans to package the device to make it suitable for operational evaluation by law enforcement and correctional agencies nationwide in 1998-99.

- *Voice Response Translator (VRT) Device*: A voice response translator device has been developed for the National Institute of Justice by Integrated Wave Technologies Inc. Belt-mounted, it will permit English-speaking law enforcement and correctional officers to communicate orally with persons who have difficulty with or cannot comprehend English. It is designed to emit an audible phrase, in another language such as Spanish or Korean, in response to a spoken prompt made by an English-speaking officer. By using the device, officers may more effectively query, inform, and direct the actions of non-English-speaking persons.

- *Pepper Spray Projectile/Disperser*: The National Institute of Justice, through Delta Defense, is finalizing the design, analysis, and testing of an improved, less-than-lethal projectile capable of dispersing the incapacitating agent oleoresin capsicum (pepper spray) launched from a standoff position. It can be used in hostage, barricade, and tactical assault situations. Specifications include a 100-foot minimum launch range, nonlethal at the minimum operational range of 50 feet, and deliverance of a fine, atomized spray of liquid pepper spray sufficient to fill a 900-cubic-foot room.

- *Laser Dazzler*: The National Institute of Justice and the Defense Advanced Research Projects Agency, through the Joint Program Steering Group, has funded LE Systems Inc. to develop a handheld device that uses a random-flashing green laser light to disorient and distract a subject. The aperture currently is being evaluated for eye-safety certification. Design configuration is like a flashlight.
- *Telemedicine*: The National Institute of Justice and the Joint Program Steering Group, in collaboration with the Bureau of Prisons and the Department of Veterans Affairs, is sponsoring a project to demonstrate and evaluate the use of telecommunications technology in the provision of medical care in a correctional environment. Telemedicine enables remote diagnosis of inmates by enabling them to be seen by medical specialists without having to be transported out of the correctional facility. It offers the potential to reduce costs and improve public safety, while providing inmates with effective health care.

State Agencies

Almost all of the fifty states have websites sponsored by their correctional services departments. You could look up each one on the internet using a common search engine such as AltaVista or Yahoo. Or, you could visit a corrections-related website and look for "links," which are the internet addresses for those websites. JUSTNET maintains a current list of links to many corrections-related websites. Exploring these sites provides excellent insight into programs and initiatives at the state level.

- The New York State Commission of Correction at http://crisny.org/government/ny/nysscoc/index.html. The Commission of Correction oversees the operation of all state and local correctional facilities. Its site includes information on its organization and history, its New Institutions Transition Assistance Program, inmate population statistics, and other related sites such as the one initiated by the New York Department of Correctional Services, at http: //www.docs.state.ny.us.
- The Ohio Department of Rehabilitation and Correction, at http://www.drc.ohio.gov/, includes information on the Department's parole and community services, business, victim services, and publications.
- The website for the Florida Department of Corrections, at http://www.dc.state.fl.us/, provides information on frequently asked questions, misconceptions, its offender network, statistics, and the latest news.

- The California Department of Corrections, at http://www.cdc. state.ca.us/, offers information on recent news releases, programs, issues and insight, as well as technology evaluation, testing, and review.

Business-Related Sites

It is increasingly common to find manufacturers who use websites to showcase their products and services. Some business concerns also provide excellent resources for the corrections practitioner.

- Jail.Net, at http://www.jail.net/, provides information and resources on correctional products and services.
- The Corrections Connection—commonly known as corrections.com at http://www.corrections.com/, is a resource that each practitioner should have bookmarked in his or her web browser. The Corrections Connection bills itself as the largest online resource for new information in corrections. This site provides links to state and federal agencies, maintains a corrections "yellow pages," contains a bid center and keeps an updated technology page.
- The American Correctional Association, at http://www.corrections.com/ aca, provides another excellent source of information on membership, conferences, publications, as well as links for corrections practitioners.
- The American Jail Association at http://www.corrections.com/aja, offers information on conferences, training, and publications for jail practitioners.

As you can see, there are many resources for corrections practitioners on the internet. The key is finding them. It is sometimes easy to get lost, but do not get frustrated. Just keep looking and exploring. The internet is one of your best resources for information on technology and a host of other topics.

∼

Dave Hart is the information services coordinator for the National Law Enforcement and Corrections Technology Center in Rockville, Maryland. Garry Pate is a corrections specialist for the National Law Enforcement and Corrections Technology Center in Rockville, Maryland.

Evaluating Correctional Technology:

What to Look for When Purchasing Perimeter Security, Communications, or Monitoring and Surveillance Systems

By Kevin Jackson

Over the last decade, technological innovation has spurred the development of new devices to improve efficiency in correctional institutions. Technological advances encompass many areas, and have led to changing roles for corrections personnel. Management information systems have been introduced as a more affordable and comprehensive means of tracking inmate activities. Perimeter security has advanced from reliance on the human observer to comprehensive electronic sensing devices.

Similar innovations have occurred in internal security—advanced X-ray devices, closed-circuit monitoring, magnetic "friskers," and officer tracking/alerting systems. Drug and alcohol abuse testing packages, telemedicine, and videoconferencing all are products of advanced technology. This technological explosion has not, however, been accompanied by a system for evaluating the utility of the advancements nor their potential impact on an agency.

Agencies are most likely to experience expanded uses of technology in the areas of perimeter security, communications, and monitoring and surveillance systems. Below, we examine each of these types of technology and provide guidelines on evaluating their efficacy for a particular agency.

Perimeter Security

A correctional facility is only as secure as its perimeter. The basic role of a perimeter security system is fourfold: deter, detect, document and deny/delay any intrusion into the protected area or facility. Six factors typically affect the probability of detection of most area surveillance sensors, although to varying degrees. These are: 1) the amount and pattern of emitted energy; 2) the size of the object; 3) distance to the object; 4) speed of the object; 5) direction of movement; and 6) reflection and absorption characteristics of the energy waves by the intruder and the environment (for example, open or wooded area, or shrubbery).

The application of security measures should be tailored to the needs and requirements of the facility to be secured. The security approach will be influenced by the type of facility or material to be protected, the nature of the environment, the client's previous security experience and any perceived threat. These perceptions form the basis for the user's initial judgment; however, they rarely are sufficient to develop an effective security posture. The nature and tempo of activity in and around the site or facility; the physical configuration of the facility to be secured; the surrounding natural and human environment; fluctuations and variations in the weather; and new or proven technologies all are factors that should be considered when planning a security system.

Some examples of intrusion-detection sensor technologies include:
- *Photo Electric Beam*—A photo electric beam transmits a beam of infrared light to a remote receiver, creating an "electronic fence." The sensors often are used to "cover" openings such as doorways or hallways, acting essentially as a trip wire. Once the beam is broken or interrupted, an alarm is generated.
- *Microwave Sensors*—These are motion-detection devices that flood a designated area with an electronic field. A movement in the zone disturbs the field and sets off an alarm. Microwave sensors may be used in exterior and interior applications.
- *Wall Vibrations*—Vibration sensors are designed to be mounted on walls, ceilings, and floors and intended to detect mechanical vibrations caused by chopping, sawing, drilling, ramming, or any type of physical-intrusion attempt that would penetrate the structure on which it is mounted.
- *Fiber Optic Wall*—A fiber optic wire sensor is in an open mesh network (quilt) applique that can be applied directly to an existing wall or roof, or installed in a wall (or roof) as it is being constructed. The fiber optic network is designed to detect the low-frequency energy (vibrations) caused by chopping, sawing, drilling, ramming, or physical attempts to penetrate the structure on which it is mounted.

- *Audio Sensors*—Audio detectors listen for noises generated by an intruder's entry into a protected area, and generally are used in internal applications, from an entrance foyer to critical data/resource storage areas.
- *Passive Ultrasonic*—This motion-detection device "listens" for ultrasonic sound energy in a protected area and reacts to high frequencies associated with intrusion attempts.
- *Active Ultrasonic*—This motion-detection device emits ultrasonic sound energy into a monitored area and reacts to a change in the reflected energy pattern.
- *Passive Infrared*—These sensors are passive; that is, they do not emit a signal. The sensor head simply registers an impulse when received. The sensor head typically is divided into several sectors, each defined with specific boundaries. Detection occurs when an emitting heat source (thermal energy) crosses two adjacent sector boundaries or crosses the same boundary twice within a specified time.
- *Interior Active Infrared*—Interior active infrared sensors generate a certain pattern of modulated infrared energy and react to a change in the modulation of the frequency or an interruption in the received energy. Both of these occurrences happen when an intruder passes through the protection zone.
- *Exterior Active Infrared*—Exterior active infrared sensors generate a multiple beam pattern of modulated infrared energy and react to a change in the modulation of the frequency or an interruption in the received energy. Both of these occurrences happen when an intruder passes through the area covered by the beams.
- *Dual-technology Passive Infrared/Microwave*—These sensors use a combination of microwave and passive-infrared technology to provide a lower false alarm rate than either of the sensors independently. This category of sensors typically is referred to as *dual-tech.*
- *Electric Field*—Electric field sensors generate an electrostatic field between and around an array of wire conductors and an electrical ground. Sensors in the system detect changes or distortion in the field. This can be caused by anyone approaching or touching the field.
- *Electrified Fence*—Positioned between double perimeter fences, an electrified fence serves as an unstaffed lethal barrier or deterrent. It consists of galvanized posts spaced approximately thirty feet apart supporting wires powered with high voltage. It is located approximately ten feet from the outer perimeter fence and approximately fifteen feet from the inner perimeter field.

- *Capacitance*—These sensors detect changes in an electrostatic field created by an array of wires installed on the top of a fence. A low-voltage signal is induced in the wire array, creating an electrical field with the fence serving as the electrical ground. A sensor processor continually measures the differential capacitance between the sensing wires and the ground. Once a change in the signal is detected at the processor, a filter screens the signal and allows signals which meet the parameters deemed characteristic of an intruder to be forwarded. When this occurs, an alarm signal is generated.
- *Strain Sensitive Cable*—Three line sensors use electric energy as a transmission-and detection-medium. The sensors maintain uniform sensitivity over the entire length of the protection zone. The cable runs from the signal processor to an end-of-line resistor, which guards against cutting, shorting, or removing the cable from the processor.
- *Fiber Optic Fence*—Light is used rather than electricity for transmission and detection. Optical fiber is a fine, strong strand of glass or other optical medium. The optical fiber guides light waves from a light source at one end to a detector at the other end of the fiber. In operation, light is pulsed through the fiber in a manner similar to an electric signal through a wire. Fiber optics, however, offer several distinct advantages over other conductive materials. Optical fiber is immune to electrical interference and electrical magnetic interference disruption. It is intrinsically safe and uses very stable equipment, making it highly reliable overall. Depending on the processor used, two basic types of fiber optic sensors can be employed: fiber optic continuity, which requires the fiber optic strand to be broken to initiate an intrusion alarm; and fiber optic microbending, which detects alterations in the light pattern caused by movement of the fiber optical cable.
- *Taut Wire*—The taut wire sensor is a series of micro-switches connected to tensioned barbed wire installed on the top of a chain-link fence or installed as the fence itself. The sensors detect changes in tension on the fence fabric. Taut wire sensors are used to protect perimeter fence lines. These are very reliable, and provide a high probability of detection and an extremely low false alarm rate. They are one of the most expensive fence sensor systems because of the laborious installation and maintenance time required.
- *In-Ground Fiber Optic*—Fiber optic sensors can be used as an in-ground, pressure-sensitive detection system. The system contains an electro-optics unit, which transmits light using an LED for the light

source. The light travels through the fiber optic and is picked up by the detector, which is very sensitive to alterations in the transmission caused by vibration and strain in the burial medium caused by walking, running, jumping, or crawling. When an adequate alteration in the light pattern takes place, an alarm signal is generated.

- *Ported Coax Buried Line*—Ported coax buried-line sensors are coaxial cables that have small, closely spaced holes in the outer shield. These openings allow electromagnetic energy to escape and radiate a short distance. Emissions from these cables create an electric field that is disturbed when an intruder enters the field. When an intrusion is attempted, the pulse signature changes radically and is picked up by the signal processor. If the variation falls outside allowable parameters, an alarm signal is generated.

- *Video Motion Detection*—These image sensors use closed circuit television (CCTV) systems to provide both an intrusion-detection capability and a means for security personnel to immediately and safely assess alarms (possible intrusions). CCTV systems offer the added benefit of documenting the events of an intrusion and the characteristics of the intruder. Video-motion detection sensors detect changes in the monitored area by comparing the "current" scene with a prerecorded "stable" scene of the area. Video motion detectors monitor the video signal being transmitted from the camera. When a change in the signal is received indicating an alteration in the image composition caused by some sort of movement in the field of surveillance, an alarm is generated and the intrusion scene is displayed at the monitoring station.

- *Radar*—This is an active sensor that has undergone substantial refinement and enhancement since its first operational use as a detection sensor in the early 1940s. Radar uses ultra-high frequency radio waves to detect intrusion of a monitored area. The radar signal "bounces" off objects in the detection zone and the reflected signal then is analyzed by a processor to determine the relative size and distance of the object. The information then is converted to symbols and displayed as part of an integrated presentation.

- *Acoustic Detection*—Acoustic air turbulence sensors detect low frequencies created by helicopters that are in their final landing phase or at close range (one to two miles). These sensors "listen" for basic sound pressure waves generated by helicopter rotor blades. Once frequencies are detected, the acoustic air-turbulence sensor sends the signal to a processor that filters out frequencies not associated with helicopter flight. If the signal passes through the narrow acoustic band filter, an alarm signal is generated. This sensor can be useful in detecting helicopter-borne intrusion attempts, which otherwise would bypass normal perimeter sensors (fence and in-ground).

Ideally, before any decisions are made about perimeter security systems, agencies should familiarize themselves with the advantages and disadvantages of each option and apply these considerations to their own sites. Each factor should be weighed in light of the demands it makes on staff time and its relative importance in maintaining security. Only after there is a clear understanding of what each system has to offer to a given facility should the choice of perimeter technology be made.

One of the factors to be considered is ease of maintenance. The new technology must be compared with the maintenance demands of the existing system. This is best done by establishing a routine, written maintenance schedule. Routine preventive maintenance will warn of problems early enough to secure parts and make adjustments before the zone or the system becomes inoperable. Also, a written log will establish the criteria against which to measure technology to be purchased.

Any plan for preventing problems ideally will include programs that not only maintain equipment, but also train staff in operating the system. Scheduled training, including refresher courses and regular equipment checks, will help keep all perimeter zones functioning.

The following issues should be considered when evaluating a perimeter security system:
1. Determine the hazards or risks to the facility's perimeter.
2. Consider relevant environmental factors when planning for a new or upgraded perimeter system.
3. Determine which perimeter technology is least susceptible to the particular environmental factors present at the facility.
4. Contact other users of the equipment to learn its weaknesses and strengths.
5. Include in the planning process considerations regarding redundancy so that weak points in one system will be covered by another technology. Ensure that the systems being installed are integrated with existing ones.

6. Examine the size of the perimeter security zones. (Smaller is better because it is easier to localize alarms, speed up response and minimize interruption of the facility's operations.)
7. Purchase equipment for which parts are readily available and will remain available, once the system is installed, and for which there are local contractors who can provide twenty-four-hour service.
8. Determine whether the facility has the appropriate electrical wiring for the system being considered.
9. Determine if the system has a good warranty — one that is explicit about what is covered.
10. Consider if the system will meet the facility's projected needs for the next five years.
11. Check plans for perimeter-security system installation prior to installation.
12. Have a trained staff member monitor installation to ensure that the installers are properly trained and working appropriately.
13. Plan to conduct defeat-testing of the system, postinstallation, in situations that simulate actual operations.
14. Ensure that the installer, vendor and/or manufacturer are under a performance bond. Determine how the bond will be enforced in the event there are problems with the system.
15. Have the vendor provide detailed drawings of the system after it is in place to simplify maintenance and repair.
16. Obtain schedules for maintenance and repair from the manufacturer, vendor and/or installer and a description of appropriate testing methods and a schedule for their use.
17. Determine if maintenance and repair of the system will be accomplished by facility staff or through a maintenance contract.
18. Specify the amount and type of training required for staff. Plan to train staff on how to operate, maintain and repair the system. Try to arrange the training as part of the sales contract.
19. Plan how follow-up training will be provided for both present personnel and new hires.
20. Consider if this system is necessary to answer the needs of the facility for perimeter security or whether it is a case of electronics for electronics' sake.

Communications Technologies

Information is crucial to a well-run correctional system. Knowing what is happening gives correctional administrators the power not only to react to problems promptly, but also to anticipate and prevent them. The key to this kind of knowledge is a well-designed communications system, one based on state-of-the-art technology that is simple to operate and that will perform continuously even while its components are being maintained and updated. Some examples of communications technologies include:

- *"Smart Cards"*—A smart card is a standard-sized plastic card with an embedded computer microchip containing a central processing unit (CPU) and up to eight kilobytes of electronic, updatable memory. Smart card technology has been emerging over the past two decades and there now are millions in circulation. The card stores all types of information about an inmate, including his or her movement, medical care, commissary purchases, treatment needs, and meals eaten.

- *Personal Locator Device*—This device provides users with a wireless transmitter that is small enough to fit in a pocket or on a keychain. This capability enables staff and inmates to have their locations monitored within the facility. Applications that require multiple-building protection can communicate via fully supervised, long-range wireless transceivers, which are ideal for campus-style facilities.

- *Personal Duress Alarms (PDA)*—When their users perceive a threat, they press the button on the transmitter of their personal duress alarm. Once activated, the system instantly relays critical information about who is in danger and their whereabouts. Strobe lights, voice alerts, sirens, or CCTV cameras and intercoms can be triggered to further deter would-be-attackers until help arrives. Personal duress alarms operate by wireless signal from an unobtrusive transmitter that can be activated either manually or automatically. Personnel who are not desk-bound often wear these alarms, especially when operating outside the immediate presence of other staff members.

- *Panic Button*—This is a type of duress alarm, usually affixed to a wall in a remote location within a cell block or another area where staff members must operate on their own. When pressed by a staff member, it sends a signal that identifies the specific site location.

- *Vehicle Radio*—This is a radio communication system in which at least one end of the radio path terminates in equipment carried in a vehicle or on a person riding in a vehicle. It can function with one or both terminals in motion. These devices typically are used when the institution employs a roving patrol around its perimeter.

- *Walkie-talkie*—These allow staff to talk with one another or with the control center. Many walkie-talkies can be programmed to sound an alarm when a staff member is thrown to the ground or if the radio is laid down horizontally.

Communications technology must anticipate the possibility that a prescribed technology that works in one place may not work in another. In other words, it must be customized to meet the unique characteristics of a single site. In no facility is it possible to keep all inhabitants, both inmates and staff, in sight at all times, or even much of the time. Consequently, personnel must rely on communications technology to maintain contact.

Additionally, communications systems must be flexible enough to meet changing conditions, because in many facilities, the mission and demographics of the population change after the facility has opened. Moreover, no one has enough staff. Shrinking budgets require reductions in operational costs, and this almost inevitably leads to a higher inmate-to-staff ratio. At the same time, the inmate profile is changing. Not only are there more inmates, but some may be more aggressive. All these factors make the need for instantaneous communication imperative, preferably while maintaining an ability to convey as much information as possible.

Correctional administrators, planners, and fiscal officers are faced with a myriad of choices when acquiring or upgrading communications systems for new or existing institutions. Managers should review available comparative information and consult with communications experts prior to making these decisions.

When communications systems are being installed and/or upgraded, the following issues should be considered:
1. Prepare a list, with input from staff, of the requirements the new system should meet.
2. Consider all possible solutions to meet the communications system requirements in order to make the most cost-efficient decisions.
3. Check plans with colleagues in other institutions to benefit from their experiences.
4. Ensure that equipment is purchased for which parts will be readily available, and for which parts will remain available once the system is installed.

5. Consider available optional telephone features, such as interface with pocket pagers, group-calling capabilities, automatic call-back, dedicated emergency phones, off-the-hook alarms, call override, cellular phones, recording capabilities, monitoring features, and hearing-aid compatibility. Also consider the following:
   - Whether the intercom network should be part of the telephone system or separate
   - Whether to use the telephone system for paging
   - Whether certain numbers should be blocked so that inmates cannot dial them
   - Where in the facility the telephones should be installed

6. Check with phone companies regarding possible profit-sharing plans.

7. Determine the number of inmate telephones needed in relation to the size of the population.

8. Develop telephone procedures to reduce the likelihood of fraudulent use by inmates.

9. Take into consideration environmental factors that may affect a radio system's effectiveness, such as the following:
   - Configuration of the buildings
   - The amount of metal in the buildings
   - Obstacles that might affect clear transmissions (trees, hills, and so forth)
   - Nearby institutions that might be using the same radio frequencies
   - Long transmission distances that may require powerful radios
   - Potential blind spots that may require extra wiring or antennas for clear transmission

10. Consider battery life and recharging capabilities for walkie-talkie radios.

11. When determining the number of walkie-talkies to be purchased, consider the need for back-ups when radios are being recharged and/or repaired.

12. Develop accountability procedures for signing out communications equipment.

13. Consider audio monitoring as part of the housing units' intercom system.

14. Ensure speakers are installed to be easily heard but out of reach of inmate tampering.

15. Check plans for communication system installations using realistic, simulated situations prior to activation.

16. Ensure that the various systems being installed can be integrated with each other. Test system components.

17. Ensure that the vendor provides detailed drawings of the system after it is in place to simplify maintenance and repair.
18. Have a trained staff member monitor installation to ensure that the installers are properly trained and working effectively.
19. Make decisions as to whom on staff should be trained to operate each system and what training schedule will be followed.
20. Ensure that the manufacturer provides a preventive-maintenance schedule at the time of installation.
21. Have the manufacturer provide a maintenance contract.
22. Select equipment for which local contractors can provide twenty-four-hour service for each system.
23. Ensure that warranties are explicit about what is covered. Make sure the system's warranties cover not just communication equipment, but transmission lines and wiring.
24. Ensure that the contractors have a performance bond, and then require the bonded contractor to fix any postinstallation problems.
25. Consider and plan for expandability. It is always cheaper to plan ahead for growth.

Monitoring and Surveillance Systems

On the theory that the best way to control inappropriate behavior is to prevent it, correctional administrators long have used monitoring and surveillance technology. The primary intent of this technology is to prevent access and/or alert staff when intruders (inmates or unauthorized individuals) are in off-limits areas and acting inappropriately. The use of monitoring and surveillance systems reduces the likelihood of escapes and diminishes threats to the orderly running of the facility. Thus, these systems help protect inmates from one another and aid in the prevention of disturbances within institutions.

Examples of monitoring and surveillance technologies include:
- *Global Positioning Satellite*—Global Positioning Satellite (GPS) receivers have been in use since the 1980s. The Global Positioning Satellite or Navstar is a constellation of twenty-four satellites in twelve-hour orbits of high inclination, containing on-board atomic clocks. The satellites are operated by the U.S. Department of Defense providing twenty-four-hour-a-day, worldwide service. A system has been developed to monitor offenders using cellular technology combined with Global Positioning Satellite. As with the regular electronic monitoring system, each offender wears an ankle bracelet, but he or she also carries

a portable tracking device (smart box), programmed with information on his or her geographical restrictions. If an offender violates his or her boundaries, the information can be transmitted directly to the police, along with the offender's geographic location. The smart box and the ankle bracelet also squawk loudly when boundaries are breached, alerting potential victims.

- *Access Control Systems*—These systems allow certain designated persons to enter otherwise secured areas. Several types of systems operate by push-button code and card-access control. Push-button code systems have keypads installed at the entrance to each controlled-access area. Those authorized to enter are given the combination to be punched into the keypad. There is no keyhole to allow locks to be picked and locks are easily recoded if prior combinations have been compromised or if there are staff changes. Card-access-control systems use card readers instead of keypads. Authorized individuals are given programmed cards that allow entrance into a given area. Magnetic key-card systems use a plastic card containing thousands of magnetic particles that are arranged to match the pattern set up in the card reader. When a match is made, the locking system is activated.
- *Closed-Circuit Television*—This is an arrangement in which television cameras, placed in potentially vulnerable areas within an institution, can be monitored by staff. It usually is located in a control center. Typical camera locations are at entrances and sallyports, in visiting areas and along the facility's perimeter.
- *Motion Detectors*—These devices use infrared light waves, radio frequency transmission, ultrasound, or microwaves to detect changes that occur in a previously empty space when a human body enters it. They detect a change in volumetric pressure or temperature changes as a consequence of radiant body heat.
- *Audio Monitors*—This technology is similar to closed circuit television, but rather than conveying an image, it picks up and transmits sound through a closed-circuit audio system to one or more locations staffed by facility personnel. Existing public address systems, with the speaker turned into a microphone, can listen to sounds in the protected area and then trigger an alarm relay when an intrusion takes place.

As with most technology, an important component in monitoring and surveillance systems is the staff who use it. System planning should incorporate both a facility's security needs and staff requirements into the design process.

The agency should retain specialized personnel who understand the problems to be solved, from both management's and users' perspectives. Administrators then can review the proposals that are most appropriate. The agency should address the following:

1. Identify all facility hazards or areas that require monitoring.
2. Determine precisely what problems the monitoring and surveillance technology should address.
3. Identify potential environmental problems (for example, lighting for closed circuit television or noise levels for audio-detection) and ensure that equipment will be able to avoid their detrimental effects.
4. Determine if the facility has the correct wiring for the new equipment.
5. Determine if the benefits expected from the equipment outweigh the costs of its purchase, installation, and maintenance.
6. Contact other users of the equipment to be purchased to benefit from their experience.
7. Purchase monitoring and surveillance equipment for which parts will be readily available, and for which parts will remain available once the system is installed and for which there are local contractors who can provide twenty-four-hour service.
8. Determine whether the system has a good warranty—one that is explicit about what is covered.
9. Develop a plan for on-site support.
10. Ask the vendor to provide detailed documentation of the monitoring and surveillance system.
11. Obtain schedules for maintenance and repair from the manufacturer, vendor, and/or installer, and a schedule for appropriate testing methods.
12. Determine if maintenance and repair of the system will be accomplished by facility staff or by maintenance contract.
13. Make sure the amount and type of training is specified. Plan for staff to be trained in how to operate, maintain, and repair the system. Try to arrange the training as part of the sales contract.
14. Decide the level of staff that will be trained and ensure that management as well as support staff are included.
15. Plan how follow-up training will be provided for both present personnel and new hires.
16. Consider whether the monitoring and surveillance system can be expanded to meet future needs of the facility.

Conclusion

The key to maximizing the use of technology in perimeter security, communications, and monitoring and surveillance systems in corrections is research and evaluation. The technology to be implemented needs to be researched and evaluated fully to determine its utility and benefit to the agency. Several states have established technology review committees to evaluate technology before purchase or use. The benefit of such committees is that the corrections agency becomes more knowledgeable about its technological needs and requirements, and will know what to ask and request of the vendor or manufacturer. Having a formal review and evaluation process improves the chances of success and satisfaction.

It also is beneficial to interrelate with other corrections agencies at the local, state, and federal levels prior to making key technological purchases. Often, other agencies already have addressed the same or related issues, and another's success or failure can save precious time and resources. In addition, ask vendors and manufacturers to provide you with a listing of their last several installations or sales so that you can check with your peers to determine a technology's strengths and weaknesses before purchasing it. Reputable technology firms should have no problem providing you with this type of information. Research and evaluation is critical to achieving satisfaction in the use of new technology within your agency. Do not sell your agency short by shortcutting this important process.

~

Kevin Jackson is a senior technology program manager for the National Institute of Justice.

The Prison Litigation Reform Act:

Its Impact on Inmate Litigation

By William C. Collins, Esq. and
Darlene C. Grant, Esq.

*I*nmate lawsuits and court intervention have been part of the correctional landscape for as long as most administrators can remember. In 1996, Congress moved aggressively to curtail the traditions of litigation and court oversight with passage of the Prison Litigation Reform Act (PLRA).

Now in its third year, PLRA has had time to become fairly well established. The early returns suggest the law is accomplishing two of its major goals: reducing federal court involvement in prison and jail matters and reducing the number of lawsuits filed by inmates.

PLRA contains several parts, each directed at what Congress had determined were abuses of the inmate legal system. Some of these parts are directed at the inmates who file the suits; others target the federal courts who decide them.

The PLRA, for the most part, does not change any substantive rights of inmates. For instance, it does not change the law about what constitutes an unconstitutional level of force against an inmate. However, it imposes what in some situations may be very substantial obstacles before an inmate can get that complaint into federal court. One dramatic example: the law precludes an inmate from obtaining damages for mental or emotional injury unless the inmate can also show that he or she sustained a physical injury. In *Oses v. Fair* (1990), for example, in which a correctional officer put the barrel of a revolver in an inmate's mouth and cocked the weapon, the court found that the action did not physically injure the inmate, but ordered the officer to pay the inmate $1,000. (The officer's conduct was allegedly in response to rumors that the inmate was having an affair with the officer's wife, who also worked at the prison.) PLRA now would prohibit this award. PLRA also somewhat limits what a federal court can do, should it agree that an inmate's rights were violated.

Termination Provisions

Among the sections of PLRA targeting the federal courts are several that require courts to terminate existing court orders unless the court finds continuing constitutional violations that justify renewal of an order in some form. The most dramatic of these termination sections require a consent decree to be terminated if the decree does not contain findings by the court that the relief imposed was "narrowly drawn, extends no further than necessary to correct the violation of the federal right, and is the least-intrusive means necessary to correct the violation of the federal right."

Consent decrees to which corrections officials have agreed over the years rarely, if ever, contained such findings because one of the key reasons officials agreed to a consent decree in the first place was that they would not have to admit to violating inmate rights. Furthermore, parties entering such decrees would have seen no need to include the recitations required by PLRA in the decree since pre-PLRA case law did not require such findings. In short, the consent decree termination provisions of PLRA retroactively changed the rules of the game for litigants and allowed defendants, or more likely their predecessors, to renege on agreements previously made.

Many administrators (and perhaps more politicians) express frustration about the requirements of sometimes very detailed consent decrees and have seized the opportunity to terminate a consent decree. In many cases, it is only the consent decree that has kept the wolves from the institution's door. For instance, a consent decree on a population cap may be the only thing saving an institution from major crowding problems or shielding its operations from very damaging budget cuts. In these institutions, termination of a decree may please a politician, but instantly may result in new problems for corrections officials.

The consent-decree termination provisions have been challenged aggressively by inmate advocates as unconstitutional. Without going into the murky legal details of such challenges—which generally question the power of the legislative branch of government to enact laws that limit the power of the judiciary—suffice it to say that some appeals courts uphold the constitutionality of the law. One does so conditionally, and one finds the law unconstitutional. The fact that federal courts of appeal now clearly disagree on whether the consent-decree termination provisions of PLRA are constitutional or not invites Supreme Court review of this very important legal issue.

Court orders (not consent decrees) entered prior to passage of PLRA became terminable two years after the effective date of PLRA (in late April, 1998). While challenges to this part of PLRA can be expected, they are not likely to have any more success than challenges to the consent-decree termination provisions.

No longer will the courts have discretion to refuse to terminate a consent order merely because compliance with all provisions of the decree would not be achieved, or if the court has good cause to believe that the conditions of confinement will deteriorate upon granting said relief. Even more curious is the fact that a correctional administrator's pleas to continue enforcement of the consent order can be legally denied by the court if there is no constitutional deprivation of rights.

The goal of Congress to limit the length of time a federal court can enforce an order against a correctional defendant is meeting with judicial approval in most jurisdictions. The days of courts holding correctional administrators accountable for requirements not mandated by the Constitution, and continuing to maintain some level of oversight for many years, may be ending.

Reducing Inmate Litigation

Congress did not limit its attention to federal courts with PLRA; legislators also attempted to address the volume of frivolous lawsuits filed by inmates. Inmates in state and federal institutions filed more than 42,215 civil rights cases in 1996, according to the Bureau of Justice Statistics. The number of inmate lawsuits has risen steadily since 1970, although the rate of increase during much of this time essentially tracked the increase in the number of inmates. In 1995, federal district courts disposed of nearly 38,000 civil rights complaints filed by state inmates. Only about 1 percent were resolved in the inmate's favor.

Claims by inmate advocates of the importance of inmates being able to file lawsuits notwithstanding, anecdotes about frivolous lawsuits, a dismissal rate approaching 100 percent, and data showing that only about 2.6 percent of state inmate filings even make it to trial, give compelling ammunition to those arguing that the door to the courthouse was open too wide for inmates prior to the enactment of the PLRA.

That the overwhelming majority of inmate cases, most of which are filed pro se, without the help of a lawyer, are dismissed in favor of defendants does not mean that a few inmate cases have not had a tremendous impact on correctional practices. Court decisions favoring inmates and the threat of serious litigation have caused more positive change in corrections than perhaps any other factor in history. The very large, unanswered question about the PLRA, along with the Supreme Court's general retreat from "inmate rights" in recent years, is whether the reduction of court oversight over correctional practices, that is, the reduction or removal of meaningful outside accountability, will permit the recurrence of the shocking conditions and practices in prisons and jails that sparked the birth of the inmate-rights movement thirty years ago.

Full Filing Fees

The most obvious way in which Congress attempted to close the courthouse door was to prohibit the practice of waiving the normal filing fee (now $150) for inmates who demonstrated a lack of funds and a desire to file a civil rights complaint. The law now requires an inmate to pay the full filing fee by making an initial down payment, followed by periodic installment payments based on whatever money is deposited into the inmate's institutional account. The law obligates institution officials to send the "easy monthly payments" to the court. Inmates who truly have no money passing through their accounts will not be affected by this change in the law, although they may accumulate a substantial bill over time.

Not all courts welcome this change in the law. A federal district court judge in Wisconsin describes the new filing fee procedures as "mean-spirited and unnecessary," (*Luedtke v. Gudmanson*, 1997). Citing the accounting burden which the law creates for court clerks (to say nothing of the prison and jail accounting offices) in processing payments, such as the inmate's initial partial filing fee of $5.04, the court goes on to complain that "Congress has passed a law that is unlikely to achieve its stated goals, [that] costs the supposed beneficiaries more than it benefits them, and [that] is a departure from the traditional view of justice."

Despite his distaste for the PLRA and despite giving the inmate's complaint a liberal reading, the judge in *Luedtke* dismissed the twelve-count complaint in its entirety as frivolous. Then, complying, perhaps reluctantly, with the requirements of the PLRA, he ordered that the Wisconsin Department of Corrections to continue to recoup the rest of the filing fee ($144.96) from moneys coming into the inmate's account and forward amounts so collected to the clerk's office.

The prediction of the judge in the *Luedtke* case that the filing-fee provisions were unlikely to achieve their goals appears to be refuted by data on inmate case filings. According to the Administrative Office of the U.S. Courts, the number of inmate petitions in 1997, the first full year in which the PLRA was in effect, totaled 28,247, an astonishing drop of 33 percent from 1996. During the first 100 days of 1998, inmates filed only 5,632 civil rights and prison condition cases, a number which, if projected out through the rest of the year, comes to slightly more than 22,000. If these numbers are accurate, the number of "inmate rights" filings in federal court will have dropped nearly 50 percent in only two years. Costs associated with processing $5.04 checks notwithstanding, if the PLRA results in a 50 percent or greater drop in the number of inmate filings, and if the goal was to cut down on the number of cases inmates filed, the PLRA appears to be accomplishing its goal, and saving its beneficiaries—prison and jail administrators, their lawyers, the courts, and ultimately, the taxpayers—more than it is costing them.

Some familiar with inmate litigation are concerned that without state legislation, which imposes similar requirements on inmate filing fees for lawsuits filed in state courts, the drop in federal court filings may be offset largely by increases in the number of lawsuits inmates file in state courts. Some states have moved to adopt their own versions of the PLRA to counter this potentiality.

As with the consent-decree termination procedures, the new procedures on filing fees have been challenged as unconstitutional. And as with the consent-decree procedures, courts consistently have upheld the new procedures. The filing fee requirements apply at both the district court and court of appeals levels, so the inmate who chooses to appeal a case dismissed for any reason faces a new filing fee.

Three-Strikes Provision

In an attempt to reduce the number of lawsuits by inmate frequent filers, the PLRA also includes its own version of the "three strikes and you're out" law. This section provides that an inmate who has had three previous lawsuits dismissed as frivolous, malicious, or failing to state a claim for relief (the latter in particular a common ground for dismissal of inmate suits) is barred from filing further lawsuits without paying the full filing fee upfront, unless the complaint includes a claim that the inmate is "under imminent danger of serious physical injury."

Courts are split on whether the three-strikes provision violates inmates' rights of access to the courts or equal protection. In *Lyon v. Vande Krol* (1996), the court found the provision unconstitutional. However, in *Abdul-Wadood v. Nathan* (7th Circuit, 1996), the provision was upheld. Many courts have simply applied the rule without pausing to analyze its constitutionality. Because a relatively small number of inmates file a substantial number of lawsuits, enforcement of the three-strikes provision of the the PLRA also may have a noticeable effect on the number of cases inmates file.

Conclusion

For nearly thirty years, correctional administrators have lived with the paradigms of extensive, long-lived court oversight and of dealing with sometimes substantial numbers of inmate lawsuits devoid of any constitutional merit. the PLRA attempts to change those paradigms and thus far appears to be successful in doing so.

The question that remains unanswered is whether the new paradigms will have a long-term positive or negative effect on corrections. For instance, that a case is dismissed by the court as failing to state a claim under the Constitution does not necessarily mean that the inmate is not trying to raise a legitimate problem, one which should be addressed, at least from an administrative perspective. That court oversight is decreased may be short-term good news to the administrator who feels beleaguered by such oversight, but if reduction in court oversight means a subsequent decline in accountability, who is the winner?

~

William C. Collins, Esq., is the editor of Correctional Law Reporter. *Darlene C. Grant, Esq., is a special master in prison-litigation matters.*

Civil Disabilities of Convicted Felons

By Susan M. Kuzma, Esq.

ou have just been released from prison after serving a sentence for a felony conviction,and you have begun to reconstruct your life. You have paid your debt to society. Or have you? When it comes to voting, owning a gun, or applying for an occupational license, an offender soon may learn that the consequences of a felony conviction linger long after the sentence has been served.

Because conviction of a felony or service of a prison sentence upon felony conviction commonly triggers the loss of various civil rights and limits an offender's ability to engage in various occupations, the reality of life in the late twentieth century is that an increasing number of people are or will become subject to disabilities, a term used here to broadly encompass all collateral consequences of conviction beyond the sentence authorized by a criminal statute.

These disabilities take many forms in many arenas, both state and federal, as established and explained by constitution, statute, regulation, rule, and court decision, and they may endure long beyond the date of conviction. While intuition may apprise us of the existence of certain disabilities, intuition is not always accurate, and disabilities are not always intuitive. Finding out about disabilities is not always a simple task, either, even if it occurred to someone to ask whether a particular disability exists.

These circumstances may explain why a survey on disabilities, titled *Civil Disabilities of Convicted Felons: A State-by-State Survey*, published by the Office of the Pardon Attorney of the U.S. Department of Justice in October 1992 and then updated in October 1996, has been so popular. Despite its rather narrow topic and, one might suppose, limited audience, the survey has become a frequently requested item, and the office's October 1996 update of the survey has been even more in demand. The increased demand is some indication of the survey's utility, as is the frequency with which the office receives thank-you letters from survey recipients who comment on the paucity of compiled and readily available information about disabilities.

Data Collection

Collecting information about the existence and nature of various disabilities and methods for their removal was a natural outgrowth of the work of the Office of the Pardon Attorney, since removal of disabilities is one of the reasons people seek a pardon. Compilation of the information was a challenge, due to the variety of state laws on the subject, the complexity of issues concerning application of disabilities, and the difficulty in obtaining current, accurate, and detailed information about disabilities. The Office of the Pardon Attorney decided to limit the scope of the survey in order to publish it before the information became outdated.

The survey concentrates primarily on felony convictions, and covers only a limited number of disabilities. The publication contains an entry for each state and the District of Columbia, and focuses on the effects of a felony conviction on three core civil rights: voting, holding state office, and sitting on a state jury. Each state's entry also includes examples of occupational disabilities and (in the 1996 edition) notes whether that state has a sex-offender registration law. Separate sections in each entry discuss the state's methods for restoring rights lost as a result of conviction, and the loss and restoration of state firearms privileges. The survey also includes a chapter on federally imposed disabilities and federal procedures for restoring rights lost as a result of conviction.

An Overview of Disabilities

Many disabilities are imposed by state, not federal, law, even for federal convictions. With regard to voting, the U.S. Constitution recognizes the right of states to determine the qualifications of electors, even in a federal election, and the fourteenth Amendment recognizes the ability of states to disenfranchise individuals for conviction of a crime. The theory that allows states to impose other disqualifications upon conviction of a federal crime is not always articulated, but the ability of states to do so seems to be accepted (or not to have been seriously questioned). Similarly, the ability of one state to impose disabilities upon residents who were convicted in another state also seems accepted.

The primary civic rights at the state level that may be affected by felony conviction are the rights to vote, hold public office, and sit on a jury. Whether considered a "right" or a "privilege," the ability to possess firearms, under federal law, nearly always is impaired by a felony conviction, and the laws of nearly all states also provide for some type of firearms disability upon at least some offenders.

Loss, suspension, or restriction of a professional or occupational license may result from a felony conviction, as well as disqualification from obtaining such a license in the future. Felons may be precluded from being bonded or from serving as a notary public. A felon may be required to register with a local law enforcement agency. A conviction may result in deportation or have other adverse immigration-related consequences. A felony conviction may be grounds for impeachment if the felon testifies as a witness. Prolonged incarceration upon conviction may be grounds for divorce. The consequences listed here are exemplary, not exhaustive.

There are varying patterns among the states in whether and for how long disabilities are imposed. The possibilities range from losing virtually no rights, to losing rights only while incarcerated, to losing all rights unless pardoned, and everything in between. Generally, the right to vote is most frequently lost but also is the most commonly restored, either by release from incarceration, service of sentence, or passage of time. Conversely, the right to sit as a juror is the most difficult to regain once lost. State firearms disabilities take various forms as well, differing on such issues as the offenses for which a disability is imposed (such as whether it extends to all felonies or only to some smaller category of felonies such as violent offenses), the scope of the disability (such as whether it extends to long guns, handguns, or both), the duration of the disability, and the method for its removal.

Occupational and professional disabilities also vary, particularly concerning the extent to which a conviction affects licensing or employment decisions. For example, some states do not permit a conviction to be the sole basis for denying employment or licensing unless the conviction is related to the occupation or profession; some disabilities may be imposed only for certain kinds of convictions; and some occupational disabilities are imposed only for a certain length of time. Typically, law enforcement agencies are not subject to such restrictions on considering convictions in making licensing decisions.

Restoration procedures vary considerably from state to state, and even from right to right. Methods for restoring rights may consist of passage of time, successful pursuit of an administrative procedure, successful pursuit of a court remedy, or a pardon. So-called "first-offender" pardons, expungement (generally, the sealing or physical destruction of the records of a conviction), reduction of a charge from a felony to a misdemeanor, and set-aside procedures (such as allowing a finding of guilt or conviction to be set aside after the offender successfully completes a period of probation) are other methods for avoiding the collateral consequences of a felony conviction. The availability of such procedures and their specific effects, however, vary considerably from jurisdiction to jurisdiction. For example, a first-offender pardon may restore civic rights but not be effective to restore firearms privileges.

Interpretational Issues

Although the states' laws vary considerably, the determination of whether a disability or a restoration procedure applies in various circumstances may raise issues of interpretation. The generalization that disabilities arise from felony convictions requires explanation, since the definition of a particular disability may not necessarily use the term "felony." In addition, some disabilities are imposed only upon conviction of specified felonies, and some may be imposed upon conviction of certain misdemeanors. For example, the federal felon-in-possession statute, generally prohibiting the possession of a firearm by a convicted felon, does not actually use the word "felon" or "felony." Instead, the phrase "crime punishable by imprisonment for a term exceeding one year" is used to define the disability; that phrase, in turn, is defined largely by what it does not include, although the statute provides that what constitutes a conviction of a crime is determined in accordance with the law of the jurisdiction in which the proceedings were held.

State constitutional or statutory provisions likewise may use particular phrases in describing the kinds of convictions that trigger the disability, such as "infamous crime," "crime of moral turpitude," "crime punishable by imprisonment in the penitentiary," and so on. These phrases may not translate well to out-of-state or federal convictions, however, and state statutory provisions may not expressly address whether and how the disabilities apply to such convictions.

Even when the term "felony" is used, questions can arise, for that word does not have a uniform meaning. What happens when the law of the state of conviction differs from the law of the state of residence with regard to what "felony" means, or with regard to whether the conduct constitutes a felony? For example, the state of conviction may provide that a crime is a felony if the legislature designates it a felony, whereas the state of residence may provide that a crime is a felony if it is punishable by a term of imprisonment exceeding one year. A defendant convicted of a crime for which the authorized penalty is two-years imprisonment, but which is designated a misdemeanor by the legislature, would be a misdemeanant in the convicting state's view, but a felon by the definition of the state of residence.

Similar questions may arise with regard to military convictions, since military offenses are not classified as felonies or misdemeanors, and may result from conduct that would not even constitute a crime, let alone a felony, under the civilian law in a particular state. Some states' laws permit resolution of such interpretational problems by providing that the disability applies only when the conduct would constitute a felony under the law of the state imposing the disability (the state of residence).

Questions of interpretation also arise regarding the effect of a restoration of rights by the state of conviction. What happens when a felon receives a restoration of rights in the state of conviction, but then moves to another state? Can the second state impose disabilities upon the offender? Can a state other than the state of conviction restore the rights of an offender? Procedures for restoring rights may be unavailable to offenders convicted in another jurisdiction, although the state imposing the disability may recognize relief granted in the state of conviction. The reasons for these limitations may be both substantive (differences in philosophy regarding punishment and rehabilitation) and practical (difficulty in obtaining records from another state).

With regard to federal convictions, some states seem to take the position that the state can impose a disability upon conviction of a federal crime, but only the president of the United States can remove the disability by granting a pardon. Their apparent rationale is that the Supremacy Clause of the U.S.

Constitution prohibits a state from removing disabilities and disqualifications imposed by state law. A similar theory, however, does not seem to lead states to refrain from imposing the disability in the first place. A number of states permit federal offenders to employ procedures for restoring rights that are available to state offenders, but for practical reasons, some state procedures may be available only to state offenders. For example, procedures to set aside a conviction and to reduce a charge from a felony to a misdemeanor are remedies available only to state offenders, as is expungement, generally.

The point at which a person is considered to have been "convicted" also may vary from state to state and from context to context. Is a defendant considered "convicted" once a finding of guilt is made or a plea of guilty is entered, or is he or she not convicted for the purposes of triggering a disability until a sentence is imposed? Must the conviction be final, in that the appeal is concluded or the time for appeal run, before the defendant is considered "convicted"? In some contexts, a person may not be considered "convicted" if he or she pleaded *nolo contendere* (no contest) to the offense. Laws imposing disabilities may not address these issues expressly, thereby leaving unresolved issues for interpretation.

Another important consideration in determining the applicability of a disability is the date of the conviction in relation to the effective date of the constitutional or statutory provision imposing the disability. Many disabilities are prospective only, applying only to crimes committed on or after a certain date. Thus, whether a disability applies at all may depend on the date of conviction. Similarly, restoration procedures change over time, and close examination must be given to whether the procedure in effect at the time restoration is sought necessarily applies, or whether the procedure in effect at the time of the conduct that led to conviction (or some other time) might apply instead.

Change Over Time

The law had changed considerably between the time the research for the 1992 survey was completed and four years later, when the survey was updated. The more recent laws reflected more restrictions on access to firearms by persons convicted of a crime. Also of interest was the emergence of disabilities for persons adjudicated delinquent for acts that would constitute crimes if prosecuted in adult court, such as firearms disabilities that last beyond the age of majority. Specific disabilities for sex offenders, including sex-offender registration requirements and occupational disabilities in fields such as teaching and child care, became common in the years following the survey's first edition. Perhaps as a result of the influence of the drafting process for sex-offender registration laws, newer laws are more likely to specifically address the treatment of federal and out-of-state convictions in defining disabilities and procedures to restore rights.

A major body of case law interpreting state laws defining disabilities has continued to develop as a result of prosecutions under the federal felon-in-possession statute. This statute defines the federal firearms disability imposed upon conviction of a state felon, in part, by whether the felon's civil rights have been restored.

Federal firearms laws also may become a force in the development of the law regarding expungement of convictions. The recently enacted federal firearms disability, for persons convicted of misdemeanor crimes involving domestic violence, has been applied to convictions predating the enactment of the disability. This disability, unlike the disability imposed upon conviction of a felony, contains no exception for law enforcement personnel, who must be able to possess and carry a firearm in order to keep their jobs and who, perhaps surprisingly, have been reportedly affected by the new law in sufficient numbers for the issue to be reported. Some affected persons have sought expungement or set-aside of their convictions to avoid the application of the disability.

Conclusion

Whether to impose disabilities upon convicted persons, what kinds of disabilities, and for how long have been subjects of discussion for some time. Both the American Law Institute's *Model Penal Code* and the American Bar Association's *Standards for Criminal Justice* address these issues. Laws imposing disabilities reflect a struggle between the competing interests of clarity and flexibility, punishment and rehabilitation, and protection of the community and reintegration of the offender into society. The coherence and consistency with which the laws resolve these competing interests vary from state to state, and piecemeal handling of disabilities is not uncommon. The result may be undesirable complexity, inflexibility, or internal inconsistency, which raises questions about the ability of an offender to comply with the laws, the ability of society to enforce those laws, and the impact of the laws on the goal of reintegrating the offender into a law-abiding society.

The ultimate goal is to ensure law-abidingness. At a minimum, that means following laws imposing disabilities, which, in turn, renders it essential that offenders be able to obtain information to enable them to follow these laws. Logic suggests that the more complex or obscure these laws are, the harder they are to follow. Further, since conviction for a crime may prevent full and equal participation in various aspects of the civic and economic life of the community, the societal justifications and objectives for imposing the disabilities should be well defined, and the scope of disabilities defined with the laws' goals in mind. Broad, indefinite, or after-the-fact restrictions on the ability of persons convicted of crimes to engage in particular activities require careful consideration and reflection about whether the rigidity and severity of such an approach is justified by identifiable societal gains in protecting the community.

Further worthy of consideration is the handling of disabilities for persons convicted in other jurisdictions. While practical constraints may make it difficult or undesirable for a state to entertain requests for restoration of rights from persons convicted in other jurisdictions, consideration can be given to recognizing relief granted by the state of conviction.

There are clearly two sides to the reintegration debate, as was well illustrated by the question a secretary who worked temporarily in the Office of the Pardon Attorney, once asked. After a week of showing considerable interest in clemency, she hesitantly said, "I really believe that people should be given a second chance. But if I'm competing for a job with someone who's been convicted of a crime, why should he be equal with me? I never did anything wrong." It is a tough question to answer. It is a tough issue for society as a whole to resolve. When has an offender paid his or her debt to society?

The price for crime cannot be too cheap, lest no one follow the law. Yet, do we achieve another bad result by making it impossible to stop paying for having committed a crime? The goal in all aspects of the criminal justice system is, through a careful balancing of competing interests, to arrive at a resolution that supports, rewards, and celebrates law-abidingness, even—and perhaps especially—among the latecomers. The way in which disabilities are defined is one piece of this complex puzzle.

∾

Susan M. Kuzma is deputy pardon attorney with the Office of the Pardon Attorney, U.S. Department of Justice. The survey, Civil Disabilities of Convicted Felons: A State-by-State Survey, *is available free of charge and can be obtained by writing the office at 500 First St. N.W., Suite 400, Washington, D.C. 20530.*

The Private Prison Industry:

A Statistical and Historical Analysis of Privatization

By Alex Singal

For years, prison authorities at the federal, state, and local levels have faced growing prison populations and increasingly crowded correctional facilities, due in part to mandatory sentencing guidelines and political pressure to incarcerate inmates for longer periods of time. According to the Justice Department's Bureau of Justice Statistics (1998), 1.25 million inmates were in the custody of state and federal prison authorities by year-end 1997, and .56 million inmates were held in local jails. A Bureau of Justice Statistics Special Report (1997a) estimated that 5.1 percent of all persons in the United States will be confined in a state or federal prison during their lifetime if present incarceration rates remain the same.

According to the Bureau of Justice Statistics (1997b), the adult jail and prison inmate populations more than doubled between 1985 and 1995, from 759,000 at the beginning of the period to more than 1.6 million 10 years later. Incarceration rates per 100,000 U.S. residents grew from 313 to 600 during the same period. The U.S. prison population is the largest in the world, with the rest of the world, excluding China, estimated to have a little more than 1 million inmates. China also is believed by industry observers to have 1 million inmates, suggesting an incarceration rate of approximately 120 per 100,000 residents based on an estimated Chinese population of 1.2 billion people.

The reasons for the dramatic increase in the U.S. inmate population and incarceration rates stem from the growth in the violent crime rate, which began in the mid-1970s, with mounting pressure over the ensuing twenty years for politicians and the government to do something to keep convicted felons off the streets. Mandatory prison sentences, especially for drug- and gun-related crimes, have resulted in prison and jail crowding in many states and within the federal prison system.

Ironically, many jurisdictions free inmates who have served less than half their sentences to make room for new inmates. However, truth-in-sentencing laws and "three-strikes" legislation for three-time felons have limited the authorities' ability to alleviate crowding with shortened sentences, particularly since Congress passed the Crime Bill in 1994. Newspaper headlines about crimes committed by parolees add to the political pressure against reducing prison sentences for convicted felons. At the same time, sentence-reduction programs used to create prison space for new offenders produce requirements for prerelease and preparole programs. According to Criminal Justice Institute statistics, prior felons accounted for 39 percent of inmates admitted to prison in 1995, while probation and parole violators accounted for approximately 17 percent of new inmates. More than three million people were on probation or parole in the United States at the end of 1995.

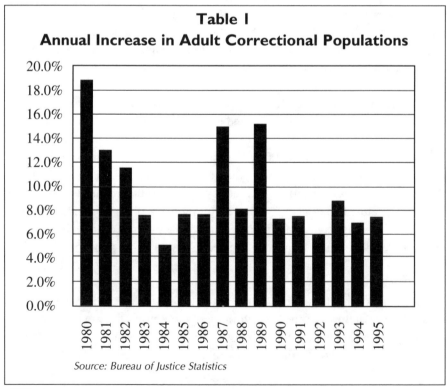

Table I
Annual Increase in Adult Correctional Populations

Source: Bureau of Justice Statistics

Studies from the Justice Department and the FBI show that the rate of violent crime has declined every year since 1994. However, what drives the demand for beds is incarceration rates. Thus, even with the recent reduction in violent crime rates, the need for jail and prison beds continues to grow. Table 1 shows the annual growth in prison populations from 1981 to 1995. Table 2 (on the next page) shows the change in average-sentences served in federal prisons for certain classes of felonies. As can be seen, the length of sentence for drugs, robbery, and firearms has grown significantly over the last ten years. During the same period, drug offenders as a percentage of all sentenced offenders in federal prison also has increased significantly. While the average length of sentence has followed a downward trend during the thirteen-year period, length of stay has increased by five months. This trend toward longer prison stays likely will continue in view of mandatory sentences and truth-in-sentencing rules.

Corrections Expenditures

According to the Bureau of Justice Statistics, the United States spent $31.4 billion on adult corrections in 1992 (the most recent year for which data is available), up from less than $7 billion in 1980. This amount represented approximately one-third of total expenditures on justice (including police) in 1992. The federal government accounts for less than 10 percent of total U.S. corrections expenditures, with the majority of corrections dollars expended at the state and local levels. Based on the growth in the inmate population since 1992, total government spending on secure adult corrections is estimated to exceed $40 billion annually.

Year-end 1995 statistics from the Criminal Justice Institute show that the federal prison system was operating at an estimated 125 percent of rated-bed capacity, while state prisons were operating at an average of 108 percent of rated capacity. The inability of the state and federal prison systems to absorb the increase in demand for beds has created a backup of sentenced inmates in local and county jails. Although recent bed-capacity additions in states like Texas have temporarily alleviated this problem, approximately 34,000 inmates were incarcerated in local jails at the end of 1995. State systems often pay localities a per diem for housing at the local level offenders who should be incarcerated in state prisons.

At the same time, many state and local governments have limited ability to raise taxes or float bonds to finance new prison construction in the face of a political environment that is increasingly hostile toward growth in government. Facing fiscal pressure on funding such important functions as education and health care, legislators are reluctant to ask their constituencies to finance incarceration facilities despite the desire to reduce violent crime by keeping felons off the streets for longer periods of time.

The Private Sector

The private prison industry began in 1983 with the formation of Corrections Corporation of America (CCA). The company was awarded one of its first contracts in 1983 with the Immigration and Naturalization Service (INS) to design, build, and manage a 350-bed, minimum-security detention facility in Houston. Corrections Corporation of America's management of this facility became an early example of the private sector's ability to provide flexibility to government agencies in operating correctional facilities. In 1987, the use of this facility was split between the Immigration and Naturalization Service

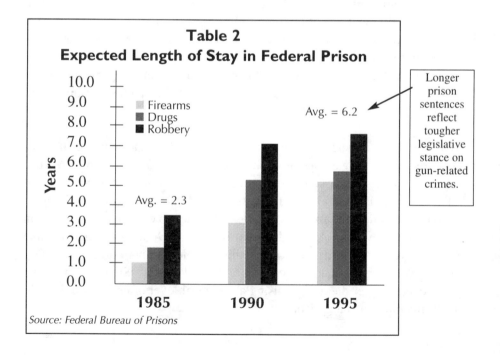

Table 2
Expected Length of Stay in Federal Prison

Longer prison sentences reflect tougher legislative stance on gun-related crimes.

Years

Firearms
Drugs
Robbery

Avg. = 6.2

Avg. = 2.3

1985   1990   1995

Source: Federal Bureau of Prisons

and the Texas Department of Criminal Justice, although the facility today houses only Immigration and Naturalization Service detainees.

From this starting point, the private corrections industry ended the decade with 10,900 beds under contract. While this represents impressive growth in seven years, the U.S. jail and prison populations exploded during this period—the state and federal prison inmate population increased by almost 276,000 (a 63 percent increase), while the jail population increased by 183,000 (an 83 percent increase).

The 1980s were thus a formative period for the private corrections industry, during which it began to establish political and economic credibility with federal, state, and local government officials and legislators. Although the industry still has opponents, particularly among some federal and state corrections officials, labor union officials, and the media, prison privatization continues to gain bipartisan support from the legislative and administrative branches of government. In addition, new prisons have been used as a source of economic development in depressed areas, with local officials interested in the stable jobs and sources of commerce that prisons and jails bring to their communities.

Since 1990, the budgetary pressures faced by all levels of government, continued growth in incarceration rates, and the emergence of well-capitalized, private-sector prison management companies have created an environment that has resulted in robust growth in beds contracted to the private sector. Table 3 (on the next page) sets forth the growth in secure adult beds under contract with the private sector. From the 10,900 beds under contract at the end of 1989, the industry's contract capacity grew almost eight-fold to 85,201 beds in 1996 (in 132 facilities, including 7,617 beds in 14 facilities outside the United States). The industry's beds under contract could cross the 100,000 mark in 1997. The private sector was awarded contracts for 21,606 beds in 1996, a gain of 34 percent. Note that these numbers include only secure adult prison and jail beds—nonsecure community corrections and juvenile correctional facilities are not included in these numbers.

Despite the accelerated level of penetration of private corrections over the last six years, beds currently in operation under private-sector management still account for only 2.9 percent of total U.S. adult secure beds. In addition, it is important to note that the industry historically has been asked by the government to manage new capacity rather than take over existing facilities. As the concept of private prison management gains acceptance, however, there should be increasing opportunities for the private sector to take over management, and/or ownership, of existing secure correctional facilities. According to the University of Florida's Center for Studies in Criminology and Law (www.crim.ufl.edu/pcp/census/llth.html), the number of adult secure beds under contract for private management is forecast to grow to 276,455 beds over the next five years, suggesting a compound annual growth rate of 26.5 percent from 1996 to 2001.

Why Privatize?

The primary motivation for government agencies to contract with private firms for correctional services include:

- Upfront reduction in construction and capital costs, and faster response times in being able to build and begin operating an incarceration facility to the extent that both the design and construction of new facilities are outsourced
- Reduced labor costs, which account for approximately two-thirds of a prison's operating expenses (Private prison managers typically pay wages that are competitive with public-sector correctional workers, with savings derived from significant reductions in staff overtime, workers' compensa-

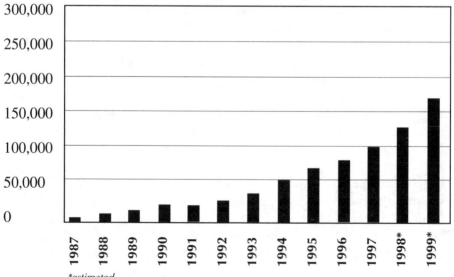

Table 3
Number of Secure Adult Prison Beds Operated
by Private Management Companies

*estimated

Source: Center for Studies in Criminlogy and Law, University of Florida

tion claims, sick leave, and more cost-effective benefit programs)

- A way to expand bed capacity in jurisdictions that are subject to state and federal employment caps
- Lower operating costs as a result of being able to buy goods and services at the best price and quality as well as eliminating government procurement procedures
- Relieving the contracting agency from having to create additional bureaucracy that is responsible for day-to-day staffing and management of a facility
- The ability to plan and control costs on a longer-term basis as contractual prices are known and fixed

According to some estimates, cost savings in facilities run by private operators range from 5 to 15 percent on a per-inmate, per-day basis. A number of studies conducted over the past few years either have documented cost savings and/or qualitative improvements achieved by private prison managers. Table 4 (on the next page) provides an overview of the conclusions of these studies. Florida is a prime example of how government can use the private sector to realize cost savings. In 1993, the Florida legislature enacted Chapter 957 of the Florida statutes, which requires that cost proposals submitted by private managers yield an operating cost savings of at least 7 percent versus the state's operating costs. The state of Florida began to use the private sector for the expansion of its correctional system in 1994, with two 750-bed adult facilities, a 1,318-bed adult facility, and three 350-bed facilities for youthful offenders.

Construction

As a result of passage of the Crime Bill by Congress in 1994, the U.S. Department of Justice has been allocated approximately $10 billion through fiscal year 2000 for the construction of new incarceration facilities. Grants are awarded to states on the condition that they implement truth-in-sentencing laws, which ensure that violent offenders serve substantial portions of their sentences. According to *Corrections Today*, top state spenders on completed construction projects for fiscal years 1995-1996 included Virginia with $337 million, Florida with $267 million, Texas with $220 million, New Jersey with $216 million, and Oregon with $175 million. The geographic trend in new prison construction is moving to the eastern United States. This is a large leap from California, which, in 1995, was the country's most active builder, with 18 percent of all projects.

Within a span of three years, there has been a growing interest not only in the management of prisons by the private sector, but a significant move toward design, finance, construction, and ownership by private companies. The increasing acceptance of prison privatization by state, local, and federal gov-

---

Table 4
Private Corrections Studies

General Accounting Office Report
GAO/GGD-96-158 Private and Public Prisons
This report is based on five studies in different states that compared the operational costs and/or quality of services of private and public correctional facilities. Studies included measures of safety, physical conditions of the facility, health care, and inmate activities. Conclusion: The review of the studies could not substantiate a cost savings from the privatization of prisons. However, it could not conclude that privatization would *not* save money. These studies offer little guidance to other jurisdictions regarding future privatization of its correctional facilities. The weaknesses in these studies range from hypothetical facilities to a focus on a specialized inmate population.
Source: General Accounting Office

Louisiana
Cost-Effectiveness Comparisons of Private Versus Public Prisons in Louisiana:
A Comprehensive Analysis of Allen, Avoyelles, and Winn Correctional Centers
William G. Archambeault, Ph.D., Louisiana State University
This study compared three facilities in the state of Louisiana. Two are operated by the private sector (CCA and Wackenhut) and the third is operated by the public sector. All three facilities were built to the same design and house the same number and types of inmates. Conclusion: It costs the state between 14 to 16 percent more to confine an inmate for one day, meaning the privately operated facilities are more cost-effective. In terms of both staff and inmate safety, the privately run prisons were determined to be safer than the publicly run prison.
Source: Louisiana State University

Wisconsin
Controlling Prison Costs in Wisconsin
Policy Research Institute Report
Corrections costs are a major issue in Wisconsin. This study compared costs at a privately managed prison in Minnesota with those of Wisconsin's newest prison. Conclusion: Private-sector management could produce annual operating cost savings of 11 to 14 percent. If applied to new prison construction of 5,000 beds, annual savings (in 1995 dollars) could range from $10 million to $12.4 million. Over the life of a twenty-year prison construction bond, these savings could pay most, or perhaps all, of the interest cost of the borrowing.
Source: Policy Research Institute

ernments has increased the willingness of private companies to invest their own capital to design, build, and manage projects.

Other trends in new prison construction with participation by the private sector include:
- larger facilities that result in economies of scale in both construction and operations
- fast-track contract awards and construction of new facilities, eliminating months from the previous start-up cycle
- the design of new facilities that are easily and readily expandable in a cost-effective manner by their operators

Who's Privatizing?

While the growth of privately managed prison facilities and beds has been impressive, the private sector still has only scratched the surface with respect to potential opportunity for managing correctional facilities. Although recent growth has come from a number of jurisdictions relatively new to prison privatization, such as California, Florida, Virginia, and the District of Columbia, Texas accounts for 31.5 percent of the privately contracted beds in the United States. Texas was in the vanguard of outsourcing prison management to private contractors in the late 1980s, as it was under court order to reduce crowding in its system.

States account for 76 percent of the inmates in privately managed facilities; the federal government, 14 percent; and local authorities, 10 percent. Table 5 (on the next page) provides information on privatization within individual states.

Twenty-five states, Puerto Rico, the District of Columbia, the three federal agencies with inmate-custody responsibilities—the Federal Bureau of Prisons, the U.S. Marshal Service, and the Immigration and Naturalization Service—and the governments of Great Britain and Australia have turned to the private sector to design, build, manage, and operate correctional facilities. To date, many states have passed enabling legislation for private contracting of secure prison management, although some states have put limitations on the type of facility or level of government that is authorized to contract. Only one state, Illinois, has a statutory prohibition against prison privatization. States that recently have awarded, or are expected to award, their first con-

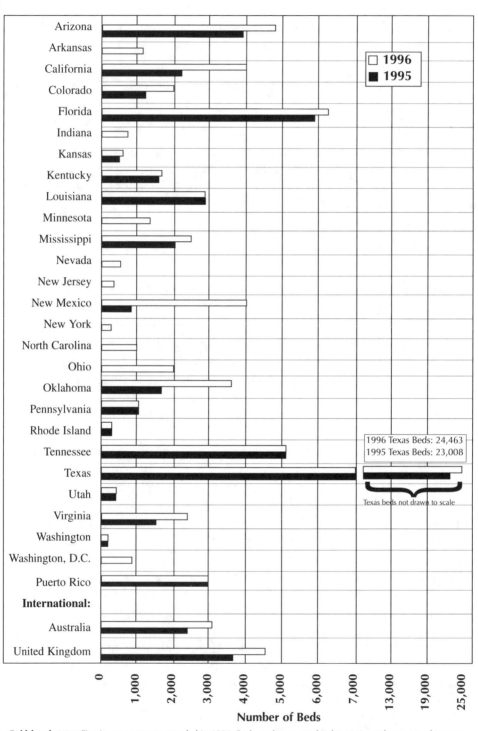

Table 5
Privately Managed Beds by State and Country

Legend:
- ☐ 1996
- ■ 1995

Arizona
Arkansas
California
Colorado
Florida
Indiana
Kansas
Kentucky
Louisiana
Minnesota
Mississippi
Nevada
New Jersey
New Mexico
New York
North Carolina
Ohio
Oklahoma
Pennsylvania
Rhode Island
Tennessee
Texas
Utah
Virginia
Washington
Washington, D.C.
Puerto Rico
International:
Australia
United Kingdom

1996 Texas Beds: 24,463
1995 Texas Beds: 23,008

Texas beds not drawn to scale

Number of Beds: 0, 1,000, 2,000, 3,000, 4,000, 5,000, 6,000, 7,000, 13,000, 19,000, 25,000

Bold-faced states: First in-state contract awarded in 1996. Beds are by geographic location, not by source of inmates.
Source: Center for Studies in Criminology and Law, University of Florida   *Dec. 1997*

tracts to the private sector include Georgia, Idaho, Michigan, and Ohio, as well as the governments of Canada and South Africa.

Business Development

Private prison management companies can take three approaches to business development. They can build facilities under the assumption that no matter where or what kind of facility they construct, the need is so great that the facility will be used. They can respond to a government request for proposal (RFP). Or, they can negotiate contracts with agencies willing to be contractually bound to using a facility once it is built either within their jurisdictions or legislation permitting, in other locations.

While these latter two approaches have resulted in a slower, more clustered development of the industry, they are significantly less risky and are followed by virtually all of the industry's participants.

The proposal process begins with the inquiring agency issuing either an RFP or a request for qualifications (RFQ). In response to an RFP, a bidder would submit a proposal describing the services that would be provided along with its qualifications, experience, and the price at which the bidder is willing to provide services. If the agency selects the RFQ process, the requesting agency selects a firm it believes to be the most qualified and negotiates terms of a contract. The length of time to complete this process varies significantly among jurisdictions, and can range from six to twelve months.

The proposal process leads to the selection of a private-sector manager. Although most privatization projects are awarded through a competitive bidding process, there has been a trend toward negotiated procurements, particularly in cases where the private manager is willing or is seeking to provide capital and own the facility.

Once the proposal has been selected, the winning vendor is granted the right to negotiate a contract. The contracting process binds together the government and the private sector. Once a contract is signed, the private sector usually is responsible for the design and construction of the facility, and often will help arrange financing.

While it has been the exception rather than the rule for correctional agencies to outsource management of existing incarceration facilities, there is likely to be increasing momentum toward the privatization of existing prisons over the next five years.

Funding Facilities

Governments essentially have two options when expanding prison capacity. Facilities with only the most basic services can be constructed, providing those incarcerated with few rehabilitation programs. This approach is the least expensive in the short term (lower per-diem costs), although many in the corrections community believe that society pays a price when inmates are released with the same education and job skills, as well as substance-abuse problems, with which they entered the criminal justice system. The other approach is to provide some combination of programs and services that will promote rehabilitation for those inmates who can and will respond to them. Inmate populations that are engaged in productive activities typically are easier to manage, reducing stress on security personnel. This method holds greater potential for long-term savings, although program expenses have the effect of increasing per-diem costs.

The cycle between an agency's decision to seek outside contractors for a new correctional facility and the actual opening of the facility (and generation of revenues) can take from six to twenty-four months (evaluation of proposals, negotiation of contract terms, construction of the facility). Given the nature of the contracts, RFPs are issued to multiple contractors to generate competitive bids. Since it can cost $10,000 to $100,000 to respond to an RFP, industry participants evaluate a number of factors concerning duration, size, potential for expansion, and estimated profitability of a project before responding. From an accounting standpoint, the cost of developing proposals usually is capitalized until either the company wins the contract, in which case the cost is amortized over the contract period, or the company determines it will not win the bid, in which case the cost of the proposal is expensed.

In the case of new prisons, construction is financed in one of three ways:
- when the contracting agency has funds available, one-time revenue appropriations are made to cover the cost of constructing the new facility
- through general obligation bonds

- through revenue bonds secured by an annual lease payment on the facility, which is subject to legislative appropriations, or through certificates of participation (COPs)

In the latter two cases, private prison companies can arrange for financing in conjunction with municipal bond underwriters. In addition, as a service to cash-strapped jurisdictions, private correctional firms can advance funds to start a construction project, thereby saving their customers time in completing a facility and adding new bed capacity. Over the last few years, there has been a growing trend toward development and ownership of facilities by the private sector, with 40 of the 118 facilities in operation or under contract in the United States at year-end 1996 owned by their managers.

Private prison management contracts usually are awarded for a one- to five-year period and can contain extension options for additional years. Extension options generally are exercised. Since the industry's inception, contract renewals have been almost universal.

Operations

After a contract has been awarded, negotiated, and signed, the private contractor builds the facility (if required under the contract) or prepares an existing structure for the intake of inmates. Once open, the company is responsible for all aspects of the operation of the facility under management, including staffing, security, supervision of inmates, general administration, and maintenance. The company provides or arranges for health care and food services, and, depending on the contract, also provides special services including education, counseling, and substance-abuse treatment. On the health care front, private managers negotiate medical caps into their contracts when possible.

Private managers generally operate their facilities in accordance with guidelines and standards of the American Correctional Association (ACA). ACA standards are the basis of an accreditation program and define policies and procedures for the operation of correctional facilities. A facility that is accredited by ACA or operated within ACA standards is expected to be able to withstand most prison-condition legal challenges brought by inmates alleging violation of their civil rights. The accreditation process takes six-to-twelve months following application to ACA, which typically is made after a facility has been in operation for several months. Accreditation has become a contract requirement in some jurisdictions. Of 118 privately managed secure adult facilities in the United States, 27 percent are ACA-accredited and an additional 28 percent are pursuing ACA accreditation.

In general, each of a private company's facilities is operated independently. An administrator, the private-sector equivalent of a warden, is responsible for the overall operation of the site, and reports to senior management. Private-sector wardens often have extensive experience managing public-sector facilities, or have had military careers. While personnel hired to staff a contractor's facilities often have corrections experience, the private sector typically provides extensive employee training as well.

All decisions regarding an inmate's detention are made by the contracting government authority. In most jurisdictions, privately managed facilities are closely monitored by contracting authorities and generally come under extensive scrutiny by politicians, the courts, and the local press. In large facilities, the contracting agency often has a contract monitor onsite permanently, and, in some cases, may have offices onsite to process and adjudicate detainees.

Private managers usually are compensated on a per-diem basis, sometimes with monthly minimum-occupancy guarantees, particularly during the start-up phase of a contract. Per diems vary considerably based on location, the level of a contractor's capital investment, and the program services provided. Contract terms generally allow for annual inflation-related, per-diem increases. Contracts typically are subject to appropriation of funds by the contracting agency.

Privatization Issues

Highlighted below are a number of issues and trends relevant to the private prison industry.

- *Prison Disturbances/Media Coverage.* Incarceration facilities, whether operated by the public or private sector, are subject to occasional disturbances and/or escapes by inmates. While the private sector has a good long-term track record, even the best-run facilities have had incidences. Prison disturbances and escapes can make front-page news in the local and sometimes national press, a factor that could result in the termination of a private operator's contract.

- *Out-of-State Inmates.* The trend of housing out-of-state inmates in states that have embraced prison privatization has benefited both the private sector as well as jurisdictions with crowded facilities. The Texas Department of Criminal Justice has begun to oversee the housing of out-of-state inmates within its boundaries as a result of a high-profile escape of out-of-state sex offenders in 1996. Should states limit or eliminate the ability to house out-of-state inmates in their jurisdictions, private managers could lose flexibility in sourcing inmates for their facilities as well as the ability to charge those customers with the greatest need for their services. At year-end 1996, 6,457 inmates were housed in privately managed facilities in jurisdictions other than the ones that sentenced them.

- *Pricing.* Some prison management companies choose to sacrifice margins on the management side of the business in order to gain market share. One strategy is to front-load compensation in the form of design and construction fees, while other strategies suggest a willingness to seek market share at any cost. Companies making low-ball bids risk providing a poor quality of service to their customers, hurting their own reputations and, potentially, that of the industry.

- *Contract Announcements and Timing.* Companies often choose to wait until after a contract is signed (rather than awarded) to announce a contract, to eliminate the negative impact of contracts that do not come to fruition.

- *Financing.* Access to capital is becoming an increasingly important competitive advantage for private prison companies. Even in the case where the contracting authority ultimately will finance a project, use of private capital has allowed some managers to assist their customers in getting facility construction started prior to the appropriation of funds or the completion of bond financing. While the private sector historically has relied on stock sales, private debt placements and bank financing to fund growth, real estate investment trusts (REITs) may continue to emerge as vehicles to finance jail and prison expansions, providing a permanent and accessible form of real estate financing to both the private and public sectors.

- *Management and Administration.* The private corrections industry is highly fragmented in terms of the number of private prison management companies, as well as firms that provide related services such as health care, food service, and substance-abuse programs. Some consolidation already has occurred, and given the large number of players and the high concentration of market share in just a few hands, further consolidation is likely.

- *Changes in Legislation Affecting Prison Operators.* The U.S. Supreme Court has ruled that states cannot crack down on criminal offenders by passing laws that take back early-release credits already authorized under previous laws. In Florida, the problem stems from a series of laws dating to 1983 that played with "gain-time" credits in an attempt to manage severe crowding in the state's prisons. In recent years, the state has attempted to reduce such credits, but the Supreme Court ruled that this may cause a problem with offenders who may have accepted plea bargains based on a sentence minus possible gain-time. This ruling, coupled with legislation that increased the rated capacity of many Florida facilities to 1.5 times the existing rate, temporarily has reduced the need for additional bed space in that state. This situation is similar to legislative changes that took place in Texas a few years ago, which, combined with extensive new construction, created temporary overcapacity of beds in the state.

- *Qualified Immunity.* Twenty years ago, the Supreme Court granted public-sector employees qualified immunity because the public sector was doing "the people's work." Corrections Corporation of America recently chose to push a recent case to the Supreme Court seeking qualified immunity for its employees because they also were doing "the people's work." The court made a decision (5-4 split) not to grant qualified immunity to the private sector. Financially, this would not appear to be a great loss to private prison operators. In Corrections Corporation of America's case, qualified immunity would have translated into an annual savings of approximately $50,000 in legal expenses. The company is still free from "clearly frivolous lawsuits." This is not the first time the Supreme Court has made a decision not to grant a private-party defendant qualified immunity. This decision has not changed any existing laws; what it has done is denied the private sector any additional protection.

- *Aging Facilities.* In addition to the increase in prison populations and the need to deal with crowding, a developing issue is the need to replace aging incarceration facilities. According to a 1992 Bureau of Justice Statistics study, there are approximately 293 U.S. prisons that are 20 to 49 years old; 289 prisons that are 50 to 99 years old; and 52 prisons that are more than 100 years old. At some point, these facilities will require replacement or renovation due to deterioration of the physical structure or because their designs have made them costly to operate. This issue could become a source of demand for private-sector prison operators over the next few years.

- *Community Corrections.* Postrelease programs have been shown to be an effective way of reducing recidivism rates. Without such follow-up programs, inmates fall back into old patterns and often are reincarcerated. In 1995, the United States spent $3.2 billion on probation and parole. Of the 3.1 million individuals under some kind of probation and parole, the largest proportion was from individuals under probation. The amount budgeted for this sector has increased 70 percent over the last five years. If the prison population continues to grow at the expected rate, the in-flow source for this segment of the private corrections industry could grow at the same pace. In the future, community corrections programs could offer good growth potential for the private sector.

- *Juvenile Corrections.* There is a consensus in Washington that violent youth crime is a real problem that threatens to grow over the next decade. According to the National Center for Policy Analysis of the Criminal Justice Center, U.S. attorneys in 1995 prosecuted only 240 cases, or less than one-half of 1 percent of 56,243 adult and juvenile criminal cases adjudicated that year. Juvenile crime remains primarily a state and local responsibility. A bill currently under review, if approved by the House, would send $1.5 billion over 3 years to states that agree to prosecute juvenile offenders as young as 13 as adults. In a national poll, 83 percent of the public agreed that juveniles convicted of their second or third crimes should be given the same punishment as adults. The effect of passage of this juvenile crime bill to private prison companies may be similar to the effect of passage of the adult crime bill. The private corrections industry achieved heightened investor attention at the same time the government appropriated additional funding through the Crime Bill.

Competition

According to the Center for Studies in Criminology and Law at the University of Florida, 17 companies operate or have contracts for 132 secure adult facilities, with 118 facilities in the United States and 7 each in the United Kingdom and Australia. Two of these companies are British companies (Group-4 and Securicor), while Corrections Corporation of America and Wackenhut each manage facilities in Britain and Australia through joint ventures. In addition, Corrections Corporation of America has an international marketing joint venture with Sodexho, a French services company with a significant equity stake in Corrections Corporation of America. Although the industry remains fragmented given the number of players in the field, there has been increasing concentration of market share for Corrections Corporation of America, in particular, and Wackenhut, secondarily, over the last three years.

At year-end 1996, six management companies accounted for just under 90 percent of all secure adult beds under contract. These companies include Corrections Corporation of America (48.8 percent), Wackenhut Corrections (26.7 percent), U.S. Corrections Corp. (4.7 percent), Management and Training Corp. (3.5 percent), Cornell Corrections (3.1 percent), and Group-4 Prison Services, Ltd. (2.8 percent).

Market Leaders

With a combined 75 percent market share, Corrections Corporation of America and Wackenhut clearly dominate the market for private management of adult secure correctional facilities. While Wackenhut is a strong number two to Corrections Corporation of America in the United States, the company has triple the number of beds outside the United States as Corrections Corporation of America.

- *Corrections Corporation of America.*, headquartered in Nashville, Tennesee, was founded in 1983, effectively pioneering the concept of private-sector management of correctional facilities. While the company struggled for the first ten years of its operation, the foundation created during its first decade laid the groundwork for it to become the industry leader. Although ownership of facilities by private operators is largely the exception rather than the rule, Corrections Corporation of America has been aggressive over the last three years in investing capital in the development of properties. The Corrections Corporation of America prison realty trust was formed in 1997 by the sale of nine Corrections Corporation of America properties. Although this REIT is independently owned and operated, it should provide Corrections Corporation of America with an efficient source of capital to fund future growth.
- *Wackenhut Corrections Corp.* Wackenhut Corrections Corp. is a partial spinoff of Wackenhut Corp., the large Florida-based provider of security and other services. Wackenhut Corp. continues to own 51 percent of Wackenhut Corrections Corp. Until recently, Wackenhut had, in contrast

to Corrections Corporation of America, pursued a relatively conservative strategy with respect to development and ownership of its projects, choosing instead to generate significant fees on design and construction of new facilities and bidding aggressively on management contracts. As a result, Wackenhut's operating margins are considerably below Corrections Corporation of America's, although the company's growth rate in revenues and earnings has been strong since Wackenhut went public in 1994.

The Second Tier

Fifteen companies share the 25 percent of the market not held by Corrections Corporation of America and Wackenhut. Two of these companies, Correctional Services Corp. (formerly Esmor Correctional Services) and Cornell Corrections, are publicly traded and have carved out positions in niche-market segments.

- Cornell Corrections. Cornell Corrections, incorporated in 1994, is a Houston-based firm. The company primarily is focused on three areas: secure adult corrections, prerelease facilities, and juvenile corrections. In 1996, Cornell's beds under contract increased 53 percent. Cornell's success has been driven primarily through its acquisition strategy, although the company was the winning bidder on one of three 500-bed projects awarded by Georgia in 1997. The company's most recent success has been the purchase of an 812-bed facility in Oklahoma.
- Correctional Services Corporation. Headquartered in Sarasota, Florida, Correctional Services Corporation (CSC) operates secure and nonsecure adult and juvenile facilities. The company's most noted success was in winning two contracts for a total of 700 juvenile prison beds in Florida. Its strategy of providing a diverse mix of correctional services has given the company a broad range of avenues to pursue.

Juvenile Corrections

Passage of the Juvenile Crime Bill could result in the appropriation of as much as $1.5 billion of additional funding for juvenile facilities. The public companies most likely to benefit from this are discussed below. History has shown that the operation of juvenile facilities is very different from the day-to-day operation of adult corrections facilities and success in one does not necessarily mean success in the other. Per diems for juvenile facilities typically are substantially higher than those for adult facilities (sometimes well over $100 per day), owing to the rehabilitative and education-oriented nature of these projects.

- *Children's Comprehensive Services.* Based in Murfreesboro, Tennesee, Children's Comprehensive Services provides educational and treatment services for at-risk and troubled youths. Programs are both residential and nonresidential in nature, and range from special education schools to secure treatment centers.
- *Youth Services International.* Based in Owing Mills, Maryland, Youth Services International (YSI) provides residential and community-based educational and behavioral change programs for approximately 3,500 youths in 12 states. The company is undergoing a significant restructuring under the leadership of a new chairman, CEO and president, Tim Cole, who formerly was chairman of Wackenhut Corrections. As part of the restructuring, Youth Services International has chosen to sell its behavioral health business and focus on its juvenile justice programs.

References

Bowman, Gary W., Simon Hakim and Paul Seidenstat. 1993. *Privatizing Correctional Institutions.* Available from the American Correctional Association, Lanham, Maryland.

Dallao, Mary. 1997. Prison Construction Trends: States Building Fewer But Larger Facilities. *Corrections Today.* Lanham, Maryland: American Correctional Association. 59(2):70-72.

Mays, G. Larry and Tara Gray, eds. 1996. *Privatization and the Provision of Correctional Services: Context and Consequences.* Available from the American Correctional Association, Lanham, Maryland.

Office of Justice Programs. 1998. *Bureau of Justice Statistics Bulletin: Prisoners in 1997.* Washington, D.C.: U.S. Department of Justice. August.

—.1997a. *Bureau of Justice Special Report: Likelihood of Going to State or Federal Prison.* U.S. Department of Justice: Washington, D.C. March.

—.1997b. *Bureau of Justice Special Report: Correctional Population in the U.S.* Washington, D.C.: U.S. Department of Justice. May.

〜

Alex Singal is a research analyst with Legg Mason Wood Walker Inc. in Pennsylvania; 1-800-888-6673. The information in this report has been prepared from sources believed to be reliable but is not guaranteed by Legg Mason and is not a complete summary or statement of all available data, nor is this to be construed as an offer to buy or sell any securities referred to herein.

Restorative Justice:

The Concept

By Howard Zehr, Ph.D.

"A revolution is occurring in criminal justice. A quiet, grassroots, seemingly unobtrusive, but truly revolutionary movement is changing the nature, the very fabric of our work."

These are the opening words in a recent publication of the National Institute of Corrections characterizing the combined community and restorative justice movements. Author Eduardo Barajas Jr., a program specialist for the National Institute of Corrections, goes on to observe that the changes extend beyond most reforms in the history of criminal justice: "What is occurring now is more than innovative, it is truly inventive . . . a 'paradigm shift.'"

The restorative justice movement has come a long way since probation officer Mark Yantzi and coworker Dave Worth first pushed two shaking offenders toward their victims' homes in Elmira, Ontario, in 1974. Who could have imagined, when we began our version of victim/offender mediation—the Victim Offender Reconciliation Program, or VORP—in Elkhart, Indiana, several years later that we were at the vanguard of a movement with the potential to revolutionize justice?

Crime as Harm

As Barajas' observation implies, restorative justice is not a matter of adding some new programs or tinkering with old ones. Instead, it involves a reorientation of how we think about crime and justice.

Restorative Justice: The Concept

At a recent consultation of restorative justice and rehabilitation specialists sponsored by the National Institute of Corrections Academy, participants agreed that two ideas were fundamental: restorative justice is harm-focused, and it promotes the engagement of an enlarged set of stakeholders. Most of restorative justice can be seen as following from these two concepts.

Restorative justice views crime, first of all, as harm done to people and communities. Our legal system, with its focus on rules and laws, often loses sight of this reality; consequently, it makes victims, at best, a secondary concern of justice. A harm focus, however, implies a central concern for victims' needs and roles. Restorative justice begins with a concern for victims and how to meet their needs, for repairing the harm as much as possible, both concretely and symbolically.

A focus on harm also implies an emphasis on offender accountability and responsibility—in concrete, not abstract, terms. Too often we have thought of accountability as punishment—pain administered to offenders for the pain they have caused. Unfortunately, this often is irrelevant or even counterproductive to real accountability. Little in the justice process encourages offenders to understand the consequences of their actions or to empathize with victims.

On the contrary, the adversarial game requires offenders to look out for themselves. Offenders are discouraged from acknowledging their responsibility and are given little opportunity to act on this responsibility in concrete ways. The "neutralizing strategies"—the stereotypes and rationalizations that offenders use to distance themselves from the people they hurt—are never challenged. So the sense of alienation from society experienced by many offenders, the feeling that they themselves are victims, is only heightened by the legal process and the prison experience.

If crime is essentially about harm, accountability means being encouraged to understand that harm, to begin to comprehend the consequences of one's behavior. Moreover, it means taking responsibility to make things right insofar as possible, both concretely and symbolically. As our foreparents knew well, wrong creates obligations; taking responsibility for those obligations is the beginning of genuine accountability.

The principle of engagement suggests that the primary parties affected by crime—victims, offenders, and members of the community—are given significant roles in the justice process. Indeed, they need to be given information about each other and to be involved in deciding what justice requires in this situation. In some cases, this may mean actual dialog between these parties, as happens in victim/offender mediation or family group conferences, to come to a consensus about what should be done. In others, it may involve indirect exchange or the use of surrogates. In any eventuality, the principle of engagement implies involvement of an enlarged circle of parties as compared to the traditional justice process.

At the risk of oversimplifying, the traditional justice approach—retributive justice and restorative justice—might be summarized as follows:

Retributive Justice

Crime is a violation of the law, and the state is the victim. The aim of justice is to establish blame (guilt) and administer pain (punishment). The process of justice is a conflict between adversaries in which the offender is pitted against state rules; intentions outweigh outcomes; and one side wins while the other loses.

Restorative Justice

Crime is a violation or harm to people and relationships.The aim of justice is to identify obligations, to meet needs, and to promote healing. The process of justice involves victims, offenders, and the community in an effort to identify obligations and solutions, maximizing the exchange of information (dialog, mutual agreement) between them.

To put restorative justice in its simplest form: crime violates people and violations create obligations. Justice should involve victims, offenders, and community members in a search to identify needs and obligations, so as to promote healing among the parties involved.

Widespread Interest

Today's interest in restorative justice at the national level follows several decades of innovation and experimentation at the community and state levels.

Victim/offender mediation programs have sprung up in at least 300 U.S. and Canadian communities. The Minnesota Department of Corrections has on staff a restorative justice planner who is working innovatively to help communities in that state develop new restorative approaches. Vermont has rethought the concept of probation, designing a "reparative probation" system for nonviolent offenders. Native American and Canadian communities are finding ways to put into operation some of their traditional approaches and values; these approaches also are being seen as part of a restorative justice framework. In academic and consulting fields, too, numerous restorative justice institutes and programs are emerging.

This interest in restorative justice is not limited to North America. Hundreds of victim/offender mediation programs have developed in European countries; Germany, Finland, and England, for example, have many such programs. South Africa is writing a new juvenile justice code incorporating restorative principles. In New Zealand, restorative justice has served to guide and help shape the family group conference approach, which is now the basis of that country's entire juvenile justice system.

Deciphering Terms

"Restorative justice" is a term which quickly connects for many people and therein lies both its strength and its weakness. Many professionals, as well as lay people, are frustrated with justice as it is commonly practiced and are immediately attracted to the idea of restoration. Restorative justice intuitively suggests a reparative, person-centered, commonsense approach. For many of us, it reflects values with which we were raised. As a result, the term has been widely embraced and used in many contexts.

But what do we mean by "restorative justice?" Will the term be used simply as a new way to name and justify the same old programs and goals? Many programs can be compatible with restorative justice if they are reshaped to fully account for restorative principles. If they are not reshaped as part of a larger restorative "lens," however, at best they will be more of the same. At worst, they may become new ways to control and punish.

All this is not to say that there is such a thing as "pure" restorative or retributive justice. Rather, justice should be seen as a continuum between two ideal types. On the one end is our Western legal system. Its strengths—such as the encouragement of human rights—are substantial. Yet, it has important weaknesses. Criminal justice tends to be punitive, conflictual, impersonal, and state-centered. It encourages the denial of responsibility and empathy on the part of offenders. It leaves victims out, ignoring their needs. Instead of discouraging wrongdoing, it often encourages it. It exacerbates rather than heals wounds.

At the other end is the restorative alternative. Victims' needs and rights are central, not peripheral. Offenders are encouraged to understand the harm they have caused and to take responsibility for it. Dialog—direct or indirect—is encouraged, and communities play important roles. Restorative justice assumes that justice can and should promote healing, both individual and societal.

Criminal justice usually is not purely retributive. On the other hand, we rarely will achieve justice that is fully restorative. A realistic goal is to move as far as we can toward a process that puts victims, offenders, and members of the affected community—and their respective needs and roles—at the center of our search for a justice that heals.

Reference

National Institute of Corrections. 1996. *Community Justice: Striving for Safe, Secure and Just Communities*. LIS Inc. March.

∽

Howard Zehr, Ph.D. is professor of sociology and restorative justice at Eastern Mennonite University and director of the Mennonite Central Committee, U.S. Office on Crime and Justice. Copies of the "restorative justice signposts" bookmark (and a list of other criminal justice resources) are available without charge from Literature Resources, Mennonite Central Committee, 21 S. 12th, Akron, Pennsylvania 17501; (717) 859-1151; e-mail: see@mcc.org.

Restorative Justice:

Hazards Along the Way

By Gordon Bazemore, Ph.D.
and Kay Pranis

*T*he promise and hope of the restorative justice vision sweeping justice professionals and community activists is not unlike that of a revival meeting. It is very exciting to be a part of change characterized by such commitment and passion. But that very commitment and passion may blind us to the pitfalls along the way. We would be wise to remember that "the road to hell is paved with good intentions," and that the journey from ideas to practice can diverge from the originating vision in countless ways.

The greatest risks identified by most critics involve implementation which fails to be true to the values of restorative justice. The values must be clearly understood and frequently articulated to guard against the dangers of straying from them in practice.

The note of caution we are sounding is based on our belief that legislation, and policy, and program changes, without fundamental change in principles and values, will not lead to restorative justice. In other words, we may see some changes in the response to youth crime labeled as "restorative justice" that have little, if anything, to do with the values and goals propogated by the greatest advocates for restorative justice.

The following lessons reflect the concerns that have emerged from our experience. We focus here on juvenile justice because we have been involved in intensive change efforts with several juvenile justice systems around the country. We believe, however, that the lessons apply to the adult system as well.

Restorative Justice: Hazards Along the Way

Lesson 1: Restorative justice is not a program. Many juvenile justice professionals seem to be aware of this now. Yet, the lesson learned in efforts to implement restorative justice is that juvenile justice systems tend to define restorative justice for all practical purposes as whatever new program is implemented as a pilot effort. Programs are indeed needed to demonstrate the principles and viability of restorative justice, but when restorative justice is equated with one program, or one sanction, or one process, the creativity of communities, victims, and staff is stifled.

Lesson 2: Top-down reforms must begin at the top. The first part of this lesson is that restorative justice reforms are not self-implementing, nor can they be mandated. Juvenile justice efforts to implement restorative justice have thus far underestimated the rigidity of bureaucracies and their capacity to neutralize, if not sabotage, restorative justice reforms. Good enabling policy and legislation have been helpful, and may be necessary in some jurisdictions. But statutes and directives alone are insufficient. Leadership and risk-taking from managers and key decision-makers also are needed. The second part of this lesson is that managers must tap the creative energy of those working at the grassroots level. When managers and direct service staff work in partnership with victims, their advocates and other community groups, then restorative justice can become a reality.

Lesson 3: Government cannot do it alone. Over the last three decades, juvenile justice agencies increasingly have been asked to assume responsibility for problems previously handled informally in the community. Restorative justice seeks to turn this around by giving victims, other citizens, and community groups an active and empowered role as partners in the response to youth crime. However, collaborating and sharing power with citizens and community groups do not come naturally to juvenile justice professionals who have been expected to function as "experts" in "fixing" delinquent and at-risk kids (*see* Lesson 5). Supporting the community role in restorative justice will require changing the system role from one of "receptacle" to one of "resource" to build the community's capacity to respond effectively to youth crime.

Lesson 4: Communities cannot do it alone. Communities are capable of active, creative, and productive involvement and leadership in restorative responses to crime. But they are not omnipotent. To be effective, citizens and community groups need support and training in the principles and basic practice of restorative justice. When this does not occur, community groups are as vulnerable as the rest of us to slipping into either retributive, or unfocused and paternalistic, service responses.

Lesson 5: Community is not a place. Juvenile justice professionals who work from the premise that the only way to engage citizens in the justice process is to find cohesive, organized neighborhoods in which to implement their programs will give up quickly on the idea of meaningful community involvement. We are learning that the most important "community" for purposes of meeting restorative sanctioning, rehabilitative, and safety goals, as well as victims' needs, are the communities of the victim and offender. In other words, "community" for purposes of restorative justice may well be the relatives or other meaningful adults in the lives of the offender, and the relatives and supporters of the victim. While community in the broader sense, both geographic and otherwise, is important in global restorative justice goals, these microcommunities often are most important in addressing the immediate needs presented by most cases.

Lesson 6: Do not design a strategy to repair the harm caused by crime without the input of those most affected by crime. Meaningful restorative justice programs and implementation plans cannot be created in a vacuum—or in the offices of juvenile correctional managers. While this may seem obvious, it is not uncommon to find programs allegedly aimed at serving and involving crime victims that have been designed without the input of victims and/or their advocates. Like any of us, victims and community members are likely to be less than enthusiastic about services and programs developed for them without their input.

Lesson 7: Address crime victims' issues first. The lesson of addressing victims' issues first is important because engaging and serving victims has proven to be the most difficult task for juvenile justice professionals. Too often we do not know what crime victims want because we do not ask them. We have learned that one of the best ways to gain the support of crime victims and their advocates for restorative justice initiatives is to ask for their assistance in designing major components of any proposed restorative justice initiative.

Lesson 8: Do not present restorative justice as something only for victims. The danger here is that staff may get the message that restorative justice is just about victim services, which in many jurisdictions are provided by victim advocates and other agencies not directly associated with juvenile justice agencies. The first problem is that the responsibility that all juvenile justice staff should have to crime victims in a restorative system becomes viewed as a responsibility unique to specialized staff. The second problem is that when restorative justice is equated with victim services, change is unlikely to occur in the way sanctioning, offering treatment/rehabilitation, and in the way of carrying out risk management of offender.

Lesson 9: Give victims multiple options. All victims are not alike and, like many of us, do not need the same things all the time. Yet, in planning for restorative justice, too often we act as if there is a generic crime victim whose needs can be met by one program. Victim/offender meetings or dialog are becoming increasingly popular in juvenile corrections, for example, and can be an excellent vehicle for victims to get and provide information about the impact of the crime (as well as letting offenders hear firsthand about the damage they have caused). But rushing to implement such a program in a jurisdiction that lacks even the most basic services for meeting the physical, material, and emotional needs of crime victims is unlikely to be met with great enthusiasm from the victims' community. The lesson for juvenile justice is that restorative reforms should begin by asking victims and their advocates what they most want and need and how juvenile justice efforts can support those interests.

Lesson 10: Do not try to fly solo. Like every other reform in criminal and juvenile justice systems, restorative justice easily can be isolated as a probation reform, a diversion approach, and so forth. To be effective, restorative justice must be systemic in its focus and scope. Judges, prosecutors, police, and public defenders need to rethink their roles in restorative reforms as much as corrections professionals do. While many of us have focused primary attention on community corrections and probation, it is, after all, judges and prosecutors who must sign off on plans to develop new community-based sanctioning approaches (for example, family group conferencing, victim-offender dialog), and it is these decision-makers who need to take leadership, with corrections professionals, in engaging the community. Like reforms that are limited to a program, reforms that are limited to one component of the system also can be coopted easily .

Lesson 11: A "balanced approach" does not mean balancing punishment and treatment. Balance also does not mean better case management schemes, risk assessment, needs assessment, and other administrative approaches aimed at improving system accountability and at providing better traditional services to offenders. The balanced approach mission, as part of a "balanced and restorative justice model," is in fact a blueprint that seeks to balance the response to the needs of victims, communities, and offenders and involve each of them in the justice process. It also seeks to balance the response to community concerns with public safety, sanctioning, and offender reintegration in a way that relates each to the other and to the overall focus on repairing the harm crime causes. Restorative justice is not about improvements in efficiency. Nor should it be sold as something that is primarily designed to save money, speed up case processing, or relieve court workloads.

Lesson 12: Community service needs community input and involvement. The lesson of community service so far is that the best way to determine whether a service project actually will result in improvements to a community is to ask community groups and community members, including crime victims, what they would like to see done. The best service projects, those that could be called "restorative," are those that also seek to involve community members and juvenile justice staff working alongside young people on projects which accomplish meaningful work which helps the disadvantaged, provides needed assistance to crime victims, and improves the quality of life in communities.

Lesson 13: Restorative justice cannot isolate itself from mainstream juvenile justice policy debates. If restorative justice is to become anything other than a few marginal programs that help a few victims and offenders, it cannot become insular and one-dimensional. In other words, restorative justice principles and values must begin to inform the way in which core public safety, rehabilitation, and sanctioning functions are addressed. A lesson thus far is that most juvenile justice systems have thought about restorative justice as a program or a process, while continuing to give primary attention to offender treatment programs, punitive court sanctioning practices, and public safety strategies heavily reliant on incarceration.

Lesson 14: Treatment is not reintegration; incarceration and detention are not public safety. Restorative justice is concerned with reintegration of offenders who have earned their way back into the community by making things right with their victims. Reintegration demands rebuilding or building relationships between young offenders and conventional adults in communities. While treatment programs may aid this process for some offenders, they do not address the core issue which many delinquent young people face—that they are disconnected from their communities. Indeed, many treatment programs further isolate young offenders from their communities and from their responsibilities to meet their obligations to those they have victimized. Similarly, most restorative justice advocates acknowledge the need for incapacitative strategies for that small group of chronic and violent offenders who continue to victimize others. But to act as if the public safety mission can be fulfilled by a sole focus on this approach is misleading. Offender-focused, incapacitative approaches ignore the potential of a range of restorative strategies, for example, to prevent school violence, to resolve conflict in local communities, and to strengthen local capacity to monitor and mentor juvenile offenders.

Lesson 15: You are what you measure. This lesson really is for managers, and it is not just about data collection and evaluation. It is about developing performance outcomes for your agency, and performance incentives for staff, that send a message that the goals of restorative justice are the most important ones. If staff incentives for promotion depend primarily on good paperwork and court appearances and only involve contact with offenders, staff likely will not attempt to work with the community and victims. Few juvenile justice managers have altered performance outcomes and performance incentives to gauge success in meeting restorative objectives linked to victim, community, and offender needs.

Lesson 16: You cannot make ice cream with toasters. This is another lesson for managers. Job descriptions in most juvenile justice systems today simply do not fit the needs of restorative justice. Restorative justice suggests that justice professionals will begin to work with victims and community members, as well as with offenders and their families, on interventions focused on repairing the harm crime causes. However, most juvenile justice systems continue to define the role of professionals as providing services or case management and surveillance focused on offenders. If my job is classified as "youth counselor," what is in it for me to work with victims and community groups? If, on the other hand, my job title is now "community justice officer," and my evaluation is based on organizing community service projects, facilitating victim-offender meetings, and working with schools on conflict resolution, I get a very different message.

Lesson 17: You want who to contact crime victims? Most juvenile justice staff are not victim-sensitive and often are not experienced in engaging the community. The danger is that mandating victim contact for staff who have no training in how to engage victims may do more harm than good. Even sensitive and well-intended staff need solid victim awareness and sensitivity training as they are asked to engage crime victims as part of their day-to-day responsibilities. They also need training and support in community development and in using citizen volunteers in the restorative justice processes.

Conclusion

Although these lessons focus on mistakes, plenty of things are going well in the restorative justice movement. For example, it appears that in trying to preserve a distinctive juvenile justice system in the face of a massive retributive onslaught, restorative justice values have been used in some jurisdictions to strengthen the commitment to the juvenile court. But restorative justice advocates today cannot afford to become isolated from the mainstream debate that is driving the increasing criminalization of the juvenile justice system. Juvenile justice systems in crisis can provide great opportunity for experimentation with "cutting-edge" restorative practice.

The restorative vision holds great promise, but not every community or jurisdiction is ready to take the leap to a new way of justice. Advocates of restorative justice should not try to force this approach on those professionals and communities that are resistant. Likewise, we should support those professionals who are eagerly taking the risks to implement restorative justice, often in unlikely and hostile environments. The new lessons of successful implementation will come from them as they work with crime victims and communities to implement truly restorative juvenile justice.

References

Bazemore. G. 1997. What's New About the Balanced Approach? *Juvenile and Family Court Journal.* Spring.

Braithwaite, J. and S. Mugford. 1994. Conditions of Successful Reintegration Ceremonies: Dealing with Juvenile Offenders. *British Journal of Criminology.*

McCold, P. and B. Wachtel. 1997. Community Is Not a Place: A New Look at Community Justice Initiatives. Paper presented to the International Conference on Justice Without Violence. June.

Stuart, B. 1995. Sentencing Circles—Making "Real" Differences. Unpublished paper. Territorial Court of the Yukon.

~

Gordon Bazemore, Ph.D. is an associate professor at Florida Atlantic University. Kay Pranis is the restorative justice planner for the Minnesota Department of Corrections.

Media Access:

Where Should You Draw the Line?

By Tip Kindel

You've just spent the last four months providing volumes of information and extensive prison access to *60 Minutes*, including two hours of questioning by correspondent Mike Wallace on complex correctional issues. When the show actually airs, however, your comments are reduced to seventy-six seconds, and the key explanations of those complex issues never actually appear.

It would be nice to think that this did not actually happen. After all, *60 Minutes* is a popular television program, and Mike Wallace a well-known reporter. But it did happen.

Many of us in corrections have had similar experiences with the print and broadcast media. Time and space constraints force reporters to condense information, and sometimes they leave out information vital to understanding a complex issue. And so you say, if we can't force the media to put all the facts in their stories, keep them out altogether! Who needs 'em anyway?

This author suggests we all do. After all, it is through the media that we are able to let our citizens know what we are doing with their money. The fact is that these are not our prisons; they belong to the public. We work for the public, and we are expected to be accountable to them. A healthy working relationship with the media is just as important as a healthy working relationship with our elected officials.

Affecting the News

Here is a practical example to consider. Tonight's television news is going to broadcast a story on complaints about your high-security housing unit. With or without you, the story is going to run. If you help the public see how the housing unit looks and is operated, that will shape its impressions of whether you or your critics are right. The public's impressions also will be influenced by a "no comment" and your refusal to cooperate. Ask yourself which response you would accept as a taxpayer.

During a 1960 presidential campaign stop in Indianapolis, John F. Kennedy was asked how he felt about harsh editorial attacks by the *Indianapolis Star*. JFK thought a moment, smiled and said, "My daddy told me a long time ago never to pick a fight with a man who buys his ink by the barrel."

Some fault the media for reporting official corruption, wrongdoing, and incompetence. But it is important to remember that the media does not create problems, it only reports them. There are those who worry, understandably, that allowing the media inside prison walls will produce stories that have an impact on prison security and the jobs of corrections officials. There is also an emerging issue of who and what qualifies as media. Both of these issues help frame the current dilemma for corrections professionals and policymakers—just how much access should the media have?

Defining Access

A sampling of prison systems reveals that media requests generally fall into two categories. One category is access to facilities, programs, officials, and inmates at random for stories on how the system is operating or how a particular program is being implemented. The other category is access to individual inmates for personal stories on them.

In the first category, prison systems tend to provide fairly liberal access to the media, and in many jurisdictions, public tours are offered so citizens can have a firsthand look at how systems are being operated. In most states, this includes permission for inmates selected at random to be asked questions.

There are some obvious exceptions. Many jurisdictions restrict access to high-security areas. A number of agencies provide videotapes of these areas instead. In California, videotapes of one of the state's high-security prisons revealed to all that it was a modern prison which was clean and orderly, and that inmates were treated humanely, quickly dispelling the negative claims of critics. The California Department of Corrections also has joined a myriad of publishers on the internet to provide information to the public directly, without media filters.

Rules vary from prison to prison and state to state on media access to individual inmates. Some states make special visiting arrangements for inmates to be interviewed by the media. Others make special arrangements for inmate-media interviews, but do not permit cameras. Still others will arrange for an inmate to be interviewed in person but will not make arrangements for telephone interviews. Several state prison systems make no special arrangements for media-inmate contact, leaving the media free to contact inmates through inmate visiting or other communication means.

Just as corrections professionals understand the power of the media, so do inmates. A press agent told me he had a media campaign planned to keep his rock star inmate/client's name before the public so he could resume his musical career when he left prison. Publicists successfully arranged national and international media interviews to enhance book sales for one California inmate who wrote about his outlaw behavior.

One inmate advocate is candid in saying she wants to promote television coverage of inmates with various illnesses to generate public sympathy and political pressure for their early release from prison. For those who have committed heinous crimes, benefits from media exposure range from increased sales of their artifacts on murder-memorabilia markets to enhanced status among other inmates. Perhaps one of the oddest media requests to this author was for a couple of inmates to provide their personal insights on the daily court activities during the O. J. Simpson trial in Los Angeles.

Another perspective to remember when determining the degree of media access is that of the victim. Many victims get upset when the offender who victimized them receives celebrity treatment from the media. Doris Tate often asked why prison officials allowed Charles Manson, the man who was convicted of murdering her daughter, Sharon, and seven others, to appear on television talk shows where he could influence vulnerable young people. Another woman complained that she felt revictimized every time she saw the man who stalked and stabbed her appear on television. The hard reality is that the media focus is on the offender and the crime, not the victim.

Defining Media

In addition to issues of media access, correctional administrators also grapple with issues of media legitimacy. Paramount Pictures reportedly is spending thousands of dollars in legal fees to force Georgia to allow the *Leeza* talk show to interview a convicted kidnapper. The *Leeza* show did not fall within the agency's definition of "news media."

So, where can we draw the line? Does the *National Enquirer* have the same rights as the *New York Times*? Do we give Howard Stern the same access as Mike Wallace? What about emerging "new media" reporters? Thanks to technology, anyone with access to a computer now can publish in cyberspace, on the internet. Should these web page publishers really be considered members of the Fourth Estate? Media organizations currently are debating just what is and is not a legitimate news organization. Thus far, there is no consensus on the issue. If journalists cannot decide who is legitimate, how can those who run the prison system decide?

The Supreme Court provided some guidance in a 1974 decision (*Pell v. Procunier*), ruling that the right of media access is no greater than that of the general public. In *Pell* and in *Turner v. Safley* (1987), U.S. Supreme Court justices ruled that prison administrators must show that a prison regulation impinging on inmates' constitutional rights is reasonably related to a legitimate penological interest. The *Pell* case identified four legitimate interests in upholding California's media regulations: rehabilitation of offenders; protection of the public; deterrence of crime; and security of the institution. One of the court's findings was that media attention glamorized inmates' crimes, distracting them from efforts toward rehabilitation and accountability for their crimes.

Accordingly, several jurisdictions allow liberal access to facilities while imposing restrictions on access to individual inmates, in part to prevent inmates from profiting from their crimes, either materially or through enhanced status as a result of media coverage. In general, the media has opposed such restrictions.

In the Courts

In the September issue of *Quill*, the magazine of the Society of Professional Journalists, Freedom of Information Committe Chairman Kyle E. Niederpruem is quoted as saying that "fighting such restrictions in lawsuits is almost impossible." As a result, media organizations have begun to use their political muscle to have state lawmakers intercede on their behalf. Thus far, these states include Virginia, Illinois, and California.

In California, legislation passed to provide prison inmates with rights to media interviews and to require prison officials to make special arrangements for inmates to be interviewed. But the bill was later vetoed by Governor Pete Wilson, who pointed out that

> . . . the purpose of imprisonment is punishment and deterrence of crime. Those that are housed in state prisons should not be treated as celebrities. Just as the legislature has enacted a ban on activities which would allow a criminal to profit materially from his crime, so should prison officials prevent media exposure that allows the criminal to enjoy notoriety at the expense of others.

Updates on particularly notorious prison inmates are believed by many media consultants and editors to be a tonic to sweeten newsstand sales or boost broadcast ratings. Often, they do. And while there are many in the media who stress professional responsibility, the current focus is on media rights.

A recent media survey sent to all correctional agencies by Charles Davis of Southern Methodist University asks whether "media policy changes are made through the legislature, public hearings, a committee system or are they strictly an internal matter?" While Davis says he is conducting a balanced academic review of prison access policies, nowhere in the twenty-four question survey are corrections professionals asked why they believe their media policies are necessary and appropriate.

Conclusion

Obviously, there are no easy answers when it comes to media policies. Prison officials first must understand what their various constituencies want. They must ensure that the reasons behind their policies are well-thought-out and that they can be clearly and rationally defined. They also must line up support outside the agency. If they then decide to restrict the media in any way, they must realize that they have just picked a fight with somebody who buys ink by the barrel.

~

Tip Kindel is the assistant director for communications for the California Department of Corrections and a member of American Correctional Association's Restorative Justice and Victim's Committees. Before embarking on a career in corrections, he spent twenty-eight years as a television journalist.

Old Habits Die Hard:

Corrections Professionals Constantly Struggle Against Negative Stereotypes

By Tim Kniest

Y ou are sitting at home, legs propped up, a nice cool drink in hand, watching the evening news, when a story about your local probation and parole office appears on the screen. The reporter is well-tailored and has a smooth professional delivery, and you think to yourself, "This is a credible person, someone who appears to know what he's talking about." But wait a minute! There is something wrong here. The reporter confuses probation with parole, and prisons with jails, and your blood pressure starts to rise. Why can't they get it right? Why don't they understand who we are and what we do?

Too often, the corrections profession is portrayed inaccurately in the news, in movies, and on television. Unfortunately, these images are the ones that become stereotypes that are hard to shake and even harder to defend. Is it any wonder that many in our profession are confused by our public image? And that no matter how hard we strive to maintain our professionalism, our own self-image is damaged by these misperceptions?

Evolution of an Image

At one time, prisons were out of sight, out of mind—closed societies that the public was not much interested in unless there was a riot, escape, or other crisis. People were aware of probation and parole, but most thought of them as supervision of juveniles, not realizing that many adults also are supervised in the community. During this period, our correctional administrators tended to avoid the limelight, and thus the media. But the times changed and so did corrections, not to mention the news business.

Following the turbulence of the late sixties and early seventies, the government lost credibility among a large segment of society. Political assassinations, the Vietnam war, and Watergate all contributed to this decline in the public's trust. The news media became more critical of government corruption and malfeasance. New standards of accountability for government institutions were created.

With the advent of these new standards came a change in the news business. Television, with its sound bites and graphic images, took the place of more complex stories. The more sensational a story, the better it was for the medium of television, and television subsequently influenced radio and print media. Stories had to have a tantalizing teaser that not only would grab the audience's attention, but also would hold onto it.

Corrections is a natural for the competitive news media market. What better place to look for juicy stories about murder, rape, kidnapping, robbery, scandal, corruption, abuse, and death? Reporters do not have to know much about corrections to report on these stories, and editors and producers do not need to know much about who we are, what we do, and why we do it to get the story on the air or in print.

Bill Bates, unit supervisor for the Missouri Department of Corrections Division of Probation and Parole, estimates that more than 70 percent of Americans use television as their primary source for news. "People like it because it is fast, easy to access and saves them time," says Bates. "People do not understand or appreciate how tough our jobs are and what often is reported is the exception, not the rule of our business." This lack of understanding by the media fuels the public's misconceptions about corrections and, in turn, diminishes the self-image of corrections staff, Bates says. "Because corrections staff rely on one another for support and assistance in their day-to-day work, morale and camaraderie are important ingredients to success. [Misrepresentations of corrections in the media] can fractionalize staff, reduce teamwork and affect how a unit and agency functions. It is to the credit of our staff that they persist in their mission," he adds.

Educating the Public

So, all we have to do to change our image is educate the media, right? Well, as Sportin' Life said in *Porgy and Bess*, "It ain't necessarily so." Law enforcement officers, the judiciary, and public officials also impact, influence, and shape our image and identity with the general public.

Mark Schreiber, assistant to the director of the Division of Adult Institutions with the Missouri Department of Corrections, has twenty years of corrections experience and another ten years in law enforcement. To this day, he encounters law enforcement officers who "do not understand why they can't bring a sidearm into a prison and, in fact, are insulted that we will not allow them inside with their weapons."

Schreiber also points out that our colleagues in law enforcement do not understand the nature of the relationship between staff and inmates. "Too often the confinement of offenders is viewed as a simple task of keeping people in cells, letting them out to eat, and avoiding contact with them," Schreiber says. This basic misunderstanding of the importance of keeping inmates busy and interacting with them in a way that promotes safety and security within the prisons is indicative of how far we have to go in educating law enforcement as well as the media.

Inmate recreational programs are so often misrepresented that it may be impossible to convince the media and public officials of their importance as management tools. They act as if once we get rid of television and weight rooms, inmates will find prison such a deprived place that they will never want to return. A good sound bite, but as we all know, not a sound correctional practice. Recreation is a constructive activity that occupies inmates' time and physical energy. If an inmate is spending time constructively, he or she has less time to act destructively. As Schreiber points out, "Recreation also allows correctional staff to interact and keep better control of inmates, because they are involved constructively."

The failure of public officials and others to understand fully the issues confuses the public and demoralizes corrections staff who feel as if their contributions to public safety are minimized in the public eye.

Changing Stereotypes

Major Dwayne Kempker is chief of custody at the Tipton Correctional Center, a medium-custody institution in West Central Missouri. He has served at several institutions of various custody levels during his thirteen-year career with the Missouri Department of Corrections and says that most of the general public, including public officials and other decision-makers, start with a perception of correctional officers learned from movies or other entertainment venues. "I am proud to be a correctional officer and proud of our profession," Kempker says. "Corrections staff are hardworking people who put their lives and health on the line in a stressful job." But the general public does not have knowledge or personal experience with corrections to know that those old stereotypes do not fit current correctional practices and personnel.

This thought was reinforced by Sergeant Dale Dinwiddie, who has nineteen months of experience as a correctional officer at Tipton. Dinwiddie worked for eleven years as a truck driver for a telephone company. When that job ended, he reluctantly came to corrections for employment, believing that correctional officers were just "guards" with little training or professionalism. Extensive training at the department's academy and on the job, however, soon changed his mind. He even compared his training with what he would have received in the military. "The training in the Department of Corrections was more extensive than what I would have received in the Air Force, but the public would be more impressed with my military job than with what I do as a CO," Dinwiddie says. "They never see when an officer puts his or her life on the line to prevent an escape or to save a life."

The misrepresentation of a correctional officer's role even can follow him or her home. Dinwiddie says that after his wife saw a videotape on the news of an inmate being maced by a correctional officer, she asked her husband if that was how he treated inmates. Bonnie Barnett, an officer at Tipton for the past two-and-a-half years, says, "We are trained to manage inmates and we can explain to our family and friends one-on-one how we do our jobs and the professionalism required of all corrections staff to complete a successful day in an institution. But we are not trained to explain to the news media and, in turn, the general public, why their image of us is inaccurate. Most COs are determined to make a mark in society and to demonstrate that they are professionals, not bullies."

Kempker agrees. "One story in a few minutes can tear down the good we have built up over years of hard work and dedication," he says, but he also adds that "corrections staff realize that deep down, the public appreciates their work and the sacrifices we make for their safety. It is unfortunate that this appreciation is not more evident to lawmakers and others because the old stereotypes overpower the reality of who we are and what we do."

Conclusion

The effect that the media, public officials, and other external forces have on staff perception is real, but can differ among employees and jurisdictions. Probation and parole officers at the district office in Sedalia, Missouri, are not as concerned about media perception as they are about how their circuit judges, prosecutors, and local law enforcement officers view their efforts. Sandy Lefevers, a seven-year veteran, says that the judges and prosecutors are the strongest influences on officers within their local criminal justice community. The more input and consideration an officer has with the courts, the more effective officers are with offenders. The result is that "officers feel more professional and what they recommend is more significant," Lefevers says.

John Mehalko, a three-year probation and parole officer in Sedalia, says that most officers concentrate on what they can control to build partnerships and relationships with the local community, treatment providers, courts, and law enforcement. Lefevers emphasizes that "if we are being proactive in establishing partnerships, we will be more effective in our role in the community and the local media will not view us as negatively."

It is more important today than ever before that each of us in the field of corrections perform our job to the best of our ability and educate the public about our profession, because, ultimately, we are only as good as what appeared in the morning paper or on the evening news.

Is it fair? In many instances, probably not. But just as we successfully manage the offenders assigned to us, we also must proactively and vigilantly influence those who determine what the public reads and sees. In this way, we can improve our standing and receive the respect and support necessary for us to meet our goal of keeping our communities safe and secure. It will be a grueling fight, but one that can be won with the same persistence, skill, and dedication we display every day in managing society's toughest offenders.

~

Tim Kniest is the public information officer for the Missouri Department of Corrections.

Index

Index

214

Index

Index

Index

Index

Index

Index

Index

Index

Index

Y

Yantzi, Mark, 185
Youngberg v. Romeo, 58
Youth. *See* Health care for juveniles
Youth Law Center, 47
Youth Services International (YSI), 184
Youthful offenders, therapeutic community,
 83

Z

Zehr, Howard, 187